Aphrodisiacs:
Incredible Edibles for Better Sex

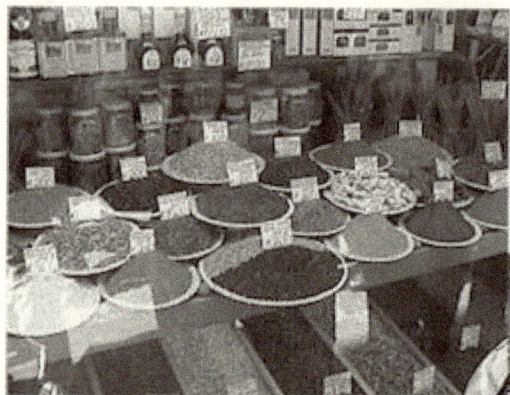

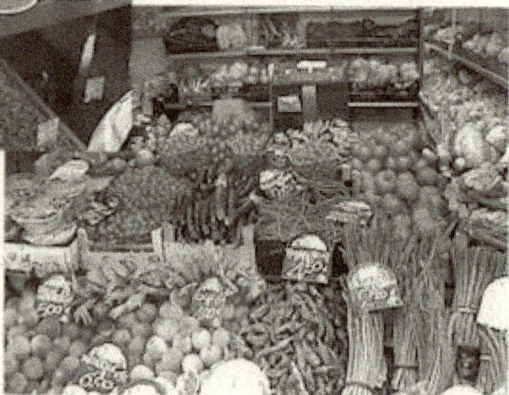

Displays of spices and produce in Venice.

Aphrodisiacs:
Incredible Edibles for Better Sex

by
Honora Finkelstein and Susan Smily

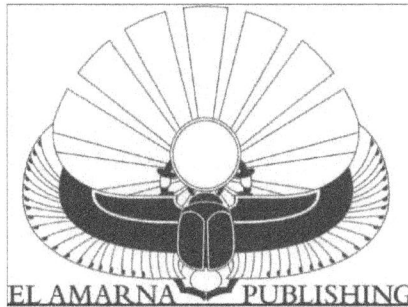

EL AMARNA PUBLISHING

Grayville, IL

www.ElAmarnaPublishing.com

Non-Fiction

Aphrodisiacs: Incredible Edibles for Better Sex
© 2013
By Honora Finkelstein & Susan Smily

First Edition, August, 2013, El Amarna Publishing
ISBN-13: 978-0615845814
ISBN-10:0615845819

Frontispiece photography by Susan Smily
Cover design by Mike Finkelstein

Printed in the United States of America

The authors and publishers wish to state that readers are advised to consult with their personal physicians/medical professionals before using any of the foods described in this book for health, wellness, medical, or other purposes. All information is presented only with educational intent.

El Amarna Publishing
Grayville, IL
Visit our website at www.ElAmarnaPublishing.com

Dedication

To people everywhere who like food and sex.
You know who you are!

TABLE OF CONTENTS

PART I: THE SWEET, SPICY, SEDUCTIVE, AND SENSUAL SIDE OF APHRODISIAC FOODS 1
The Apple of Eve 1
Aphrodisiac Foods, Spices, and Herbs 3

PART II: APHRODISIACS 101 5
What *Is* an Aphrodisiac? 5
How Do Aphrodisiacs Work? 6
Some Evidence of Aphrodisiac Experiences 8

PART III: GETTING IT ON WITH GOOD NUTRITION 11
Vitamin A, B-Complex 11
Vitamin C, Vitamin D3 12
Vitamin E, Vitamin K2 13
DHEA, Arginine 14
Tyrosine, Zinc 15

PART IV: FRUITS, NUTS AND SEEDS 17
1. Fruits 17
    Apricots, Avocadoes 17
    Bananas, Cherries 18
    Date Palm, Figs 19
    Goji Berries, Grapes 20
    Mangoes, Olives and Olive Oil, Papaya 21
    Pomegranates 22
    Pineapple, Raspberries and Strawberries 23
    Saw Palmetto, Watermelon 24
2. Nuts 25
    Almonds 25
    Cashews 26
3. Seeds 26
    Anise Seed 26
    Pumpkin Seeds, Pine Nuts, Sunflowers and Sunflower Seeds 27

PART V: VEGETABLES 29
1. Flower Buds 29
    Artichoke, Broccoli 29
2. Leaves 30
    Lovage, Spinach 30
3. Stems 31
    Asparagus, Celery 31
4. Rhizomes and Tubers 32
    Ginger, Potatoes, Sweet Potatoes, and Yams 32

5. Roots 33
    Beets 33
    Carrots, Ginseng 34
    Maca 35
6. Bulbs 35
    Onions, Garlic 35
    Shallots 36
7. Fruits Used as Vegetables 37
    Cucumber, Okra, Squash 37
    Tomatoes 38

PART VI: HERBS 39
1. Parsley, Sage, Rosemary, and Thyme 39
    Parsley 39
    Sage 40
    Rosemary, Thyme 41

2. Other Herbs (Besides the Ones at Scarborough Fair) 42
    Arugula 42
    Dill, Mint 43
    Sarsaparilla 44
    Yarrow 45

PART VII: SPICES 47
Basil, Black Peppercorns 47
Cardamom, Cayenne and Other Hot Chili Peppers 48
Cinnamon, Cloves, Coriander (Dried Cilantro Seed) 49
Cumin, Fennel 50
Mustard 51
Nutmeg and Mace, Pimento/Allspice 52
Turmeric 53
Saffron 54

PART VIII: MORE VEGETATIVE MATTER 55
1. Flowers and Leaves 55
    Albuca, Damiana, Rose 55
    Ginkgo Biloba 56
    Ylang-Ylang 57
2. Pulses 57
    Licorice 58
3. Coffee, Chocolate, and Vanilla 59
    Coffee, Chocolate/Cocoa 59
    Vanilla 60
4. Rice, Wheat Germ, Soy, and Oats 61
    Rice, Wheat Germ, Soy 61
    Oats 62

PART IX: ANIMAL PROTEINS...**63**
1. Dairy and Meat... 63
   Cheese, Eggs 63
   Meat 64
2. Seafood and Fish.. 64
   Eel, Mussels... 65
   Oysters 66

PART X: ALCOHOL...**67**
Absinthe, Agave 67
Wine.. 68

PART XI: A FEW OTHER FOODS OF INTEREST **69**
Honey 69
Kelp, Mushrooms, Sauerkraut 70
Spirulina, Truffles.. 71

PART XII: SOME NOT SO COMMON PLANTS
WITH AN APHRODISIAC HISTORY **73**
Acorus Calamus (Sweet Flag), Asafoetida 73
Ashwagandha/Withania Somnifera 73
Catuaba, Cistanche, Cnidium Seeds.................................. 74
Durian Fruit, Guarana, Horny Goat Weed 75
Huanarpo Macho, Muira Puama.. 76
Picho Huayo, Rhodiola Rosea.. 77
Rosewood Oil, Tamamuri, Tongkat Ali.............................. 78
Tribulus Terrestris 79

PART XIII: PSYCHOTROPIC APHRODISIACS **80**
Belladonna, Betel Palm Seeds.. 80
Borrachero, Datura, Hawaiian Baby Woodrose.................. 81
Kava, Mandrake Root... 82
Morning Glory Seeds, Passion Flowers and Passion Fruits 84
Poppy Seeds, Prickly or Mexican Poppy 85
Sassafras, Spanish Fly 86
Wild Lettuce.. 87
Yohimbine 88

PART XIV: IN CONCLUSION **89**
ABOUT THE AUTHORS **91**
OUR BOOKS **93**
ABOUT EL AMARNA PUBLISHING...............................**95**

Part I:
The Sweet, Spicy, Seductive, and Sensual Side of Aphrodisiac Foods

The Apple of Eve

Eve's apple was the first food that got us humans into trouble. You know the details: God gave Adam and Eve a warning:

"You can nosh on everything in Eden except the fruit of a couple of trees—this one and that one," he said, pointing to the Tree of Knowledge and the Tree of Life.

So they said okay, but while Adam was off napping, Eve was just wandering along, humming a little tune, and looking up at the Tree of Knowledge with its pretty red apples, when a snake slithered down it and said with a big smile, "Wanna try one? They're on special today only!"

When Eve took a bite, she realized she might need somebody else to blame, so she woke Adam up from his nap and offered him a bite, too. He was still sleepy, but she said, "Here, Honey, have some—it tastes really good."

"How do you know?" asked Adam.

"I already had a bite, and it was yummy," she said enthusiastically.

Since she hadn't died or turned into a gnarly old granny, he figured it couldn't hurt. So he bit, too—and opened the trapdoor to all our human woes including death—or at least, that's how the story goes.

You can think of this story from Genesis as a probable parable about how humans became involved in the sensuality of the physical plane, because eating is the one thing we do that involves *all* the senses.

We *see* the beautiful red apple. We *feel* its smooth skin with our fingers. We *smell* its scent—ummm! We bite into its juicy goodness and *taste* its sweet tang. And as we take that first bite, we *hear* the crunch.

So we engage all five of our senses in eating the apple. Ergo, the story of Eve's apple is a terrific tale about getting caught in the sensual world of physical experience—and how you tend to lose your focus on spirituality when you become so wrapped up in the senses.

Is the story of Adam and Eve also about sex? Well, yeah, probably. The tree from which the apple came was the Tree of Knowledge, and "knowing," in the biblical sense, means having sex, though whether that's what the original Hebrew meant is something I can't say for sure—I'll have to leave that kind of determination to the rabbis. But I'll grant that sex is definitely *the* most pleasurable sensual experience human beings can have.

However, as we quoted in our second *Killer Cookbook*[1], anyone who eats three meals a day knows why cookbooks outsell sex books three to one—most of us, except maybe young people in a new relationship, eat a lot more often than we have sex. Nevertheless, anything having to do with sex still sells very well—as witnessed by the recent success of *50 Shades of Gray*. So let's face it, most of us like to eat, and most of us *really* enjoy sex. And naturally, when we put these two pleasures together, there's the implication that we'll enjoy both experiences more.

After Eve and Adam's little snack in the garden, the connection of the pleasures of food and sex eventually led to the idea that perhaps foods could enhance the pleasure of sex or maybe even give one gender or the other an increased desire for sex. So, when people consciously feed other people aphrodisiac foods, their intention is to follow the pleasurable experience of eating with an enhanced

---

1 *The Lawyer Who Died Trying*, El Amarna Publishing, 2012. The paperback edition of the novel includes the complete *Killer Cookbook #2, Recipes to Accompany The Lawyer Who Died Trying*. (There is a link in the Kindle edition to a free PDF download of the cookbook.)

pleasurable experience in the bedroom—or wherever. (This is why guys buy their girlfriends dinner, because going Dutch doesn't imply any expectations afterward.)

Oh, and lest we forget, it's important to know that too much of a true aphrodisiac can be poisonous. Hence, it behooves us all to be informed about the aphrodisiac qualities of all foods.

Aphrodisiac Foods, Spices, and Herbs

Most of the foods listed in this book are common ones the majority of us eat regularly, provided we like our fruits and veggies, though some of these plant-based items are more commonly found at health food stores than in the produce section of grocery stores. Few people realize just how sexy some of these foods are, so that's why we've made this list.

In addition, we're including certain flowers, especially if they or some of their parts are regularly ingested. And we're including spices and herbs, the little jewels of the plant kingdom, which awaken the senses of taste and olfaction. They have also been used in food preparation for centuries to improve the *quality* of a food's taste.

You might prefer not to know this, but sometimes the spiciest dishes on the planet are made hot by their cooks because the basic foods themselves may be slightly rancid, and giving foods a hot, spicy taste can hide that fact and make them more palatable. In fact, spices were so prized when they finally made their way from Asia to Europe via the camel trains of the Middle East that they sparked the desire on the part of European traders and merchants to find a shorter, faster route to the Spice Islands of the Far East. So spices were at least in part responsible for the discovery of the New World.

Part II:
Aphrodisiacs 101

What *Is* an Aphrodisiac?

So you may ask, what, exactly, is an aphrodisiac? This word derives from the name of the Greek goddess of love and sex, Aphrodite, who was known in the Roman world as Venus. The term "aphrodisiac" applies to any food, drink, or other compound that might be eaten or imbibed, smelled, bathed in or rubbed onto the body so that it's taken in through the skin, or even inserted into other orifices or rubbed into the sex organs so that it can contribute to the desire for sex.

Queen Cleopatra seems to have believed in the aphrodisiac quality of good smells, so she stirred up a concoction from bear grease, opiates, and perfume to excite and subdue her lovers, and this sounds like it could have been a massage treatment rather than something edible. Julius Caesar, who *was* one of Cleopatra's lovers, thought the scent of perfume could excite all people to the fires of love and passion, and it appears Romans of his day applied perfume regularly, so maybe Cleopatra's bear grease rub was effective. (But then, Honora's mother used to say, "If you don't have an opportunity to use soap, then for pity's sake, use perfume!" So maybe Julius just hadn't had a chance to get to the Roman baths regularly.)

If your libido isn't up to par, consider giving it a little help with the essential oils of aromatherapy. When our olfactory senses are stimulated, they in turn can stimulate the limbic system in the brain which gives a nudge to the libido. At the same time, the smell of these essential oils triggers the master gland of the body, the pituitary, to uplevel hormone production. So sweet-smelling odors can get the body in the mood for sex. Perhaps this is why the Vajikarana Tantra of

Ayurvedic medicine recommends aphrodisiac smells to assist in overcoming sexual dysfunctions.

How Do Aphrodisiacs Work?

Much of the lore around the *modus operandi* of aphrodisiacs comes to us from what might be termed "sympathetic magic," wherein if something is *not* a duck but *looks like* a duck, it is presumed that it will have influence like that of a duck. So it was believed that items having a physical resemblance to the human sex organs would, when eaten, have influence on the arousal of the sex organs of the person doing the eating.

For example, bananas, cucumbers, and long, thick asparagus would be considered male aphrodisiacs because they have the proper stiff penis shape, while the widely touted oyster, which some people think resembles the female genitalia, would be considered an appropriate aphrodisiac for women.

On the other hand, it might be a turn-on for a man to watch his partner *really* enjoy eating a banana, and it might be a turn-on for a woman to watch her partner totally get into eating an oyster.

In ancient times, foods resembling seeds, such as fish eggs, would have been thought to enhance both sexual potency and fertility.

Of course, many plants and herbs are toxic, and others, though they can be ingested in tiny amounts to bring beneficial effects, could kill if they are used in large amounts. We'll examine a list of killer aphrodisiacs toward the end of this book.

While we're on the subject of magic, in ages past and perhaps even today, practitioners of herbalism might well include psychotropic plants or other substances in both love potions and lotions, and using these could cause a sufficiently altered perception of reality to bring about a change in sexual performance. Whether that change would be considered positive or negative would, of course, be up to the individual experiencing it. But it's worth noting that some of the reputation for the effects of aphrodisiacs may come from the psychedelic effects of certain plant or mineral substances used in shamanic rituals to engender altered states in order to connect with spirits and to prophesy or bring about healing. Such food or plants that have psychotropic properties are called *entheogens* when they are used for shamanic or spiritual purposes.

In ancient Greece and Rome, both of which were cultures particularly interested in sexual activity that actually made the act of love an art, aphrodisiacs were sought to calm sexual anxieties, because an inadequate performance on the part of either gender can create serious problems for a sexual interaction.

Also, in ancient times, people made a distinction between substances that increased fertility versus those that increased the sex drive, so some foods were valued for enhancing the desire for sex, while others were thought to increase fertility or male potency.

As the *Cambridge World History of Food* points out, undernourishment was a problem in some early cultures, as food wasn't as available in ancient times as it is today. One thing under-eating can cause is lack of libido, and it can also put a damper on fertility and virility. Following these ideas to their natural conclusion, if a person can't perform sexually, there's not much chance of that person being able to procreate, and procreation in ancient times was an important goal because people didn't live exceptionally long lives, and most people believed it was important to reproduce little facsimiles of themselves before their expiration dates came up.

It's also important to note as a preliminary disclaimer that most, though not all, modern medical personnel and researchers claim not to believe in the power of aphrodisiacs in foodstuffs or natural substances—however, they're perfectly happy to sell Viagra to men and pheromone-enhancing pharmaceuticals to women because these are laboratory-made chemicals.

On the other hand, *some* researchers are finding that the nutritional elements found in many foods reputed to be aphrodisiacs do in fact have a positive effect on libido, on the increase in hormone production, on fertility and virility, on male potency, and even on sexual desire. So all we can say is, if you know the aphrodisiac associations of a certain food as well as the nutritional elements in that food and what they might contribute to your sexual prowess, and you eat that food with good results, then you may just be suggestible and the results may be psychosomatic. But then again, you could adopt a pragmatic attitude and simply say, "If it works for me, then it works for *me*," and not worry about whether it works for anybody else—your doctor and pharmaceutical researchers included!

Some Evidence of Aphrodisiac Experiences

Historically, the human animal has often combined the pleasures of either eating or drinking with sex.

One of the earliest aphrodisiacs for the ancient Greeks was the sparrow, a bird sacred to Aphrodite because of its lascivious nature. Sparrows don't have much meat on their little bodies, so the brains were added to give the concoction more clout—and of course, sparrow spare parts could be added to other mixtures. Later on, rabbits, which reproduce at an alarmingly rapid rate, would be eaten for their lusty nature as well as for their tasty meat.

The Dionysian rites of the Greeks included the imbibing of copious amounts of wine with sexual activity. An actor playing the role of Dionysus would come out, all painted red like the color of wine and covered with bunches of grapes. He'd be accompanied by other actors dressed as satyrs, with little horns on their heads and hairy leggings ending in goat-like hooves. These satyrs sported huge penises and are reported to have chanted, "I am the god of sex—I am the god of love." And of course, they'd chase the attractive maidens in the audience when they got the chance.

However, as we all know, a little bit of wine can be a good thing when it relieves one's inhibitions, but it can be a bad thing—making one unavailable for sexual activity—when one imbibes too much and gets drunk.

The later Romans were reported also to have combined the luxuries of elaborate banquets with orgiastic behavior. There's a wonderful mosaic floor in a still extant banquet hall that shows all the leavings, like partially eaten pieces of food and fish bones, which were to be thrown on the floor when more interesting entertainment became available to the participants—and orgiastic entertainment was reputedly often a part of elaborate banquets in Rome. This detritus on the banquet hall floor is of course beautifully depicted in mosaic art.

In medieval times, pharmacologists would mix up powdered gold in an elixir and sell it as an aphrodisiac for vast amounts of money.

The 18th-century period movie *Tom Jones* contains a marvelous comic scene[2] where Tom and the woman he is desirous of bedding have an elaborate banquet at a wayside inn, and though no words are spoken as they gorge themselves on the food, we see them becoming more and more sexually aroused as they gobble down all the goodies while watching each other eat.

We once saw a *CSI* episode that involved a restaurant where the clientele was literally kept in the dark during dinner, the idea being that all the other senses are heightened when one's vision is turned off. All the waiters were blind or wearing eye coverings, and clients were not discouraged from indulging in hanky-panky. So the sensuality of the food could lead to the sensuality of sexual activity right there at the dinner table. Of course, the CSIs were called in when a Hugh Hefner look-alike was murdered while surrounded by luscious lady friends in scanty clothing. Naturally, nobody "saw" anything, so other reports of sense experiences besides eye-witness ones—especially as combined with eating—were required for the solution to the murder.

---

[2] If you're too young to remember this film, which came out in 1963, you can still get it on Turner Classic Movies.

Part III:
Getting It On with Good Nutrition

There's no question that good nutrition can contribute to good sex. So let's take a look at the nutritional elements that can improve sexual performance, and then we'll be able to see why certain foods are on the aphrodisiac list of "good performers."

Vitamin A

Vitamin A is essential for healthy sexual reproduction. A deficiency of this vitamin in research studies has caused atrophy of the sex organs of rats, leaving them sterilized. Since sex hormones are necessary for healthy skin, it is believed there's a correlation between having skin that's dry and scaly and a deficiency of this vitamin, which is plentiful in fish and eggs, cheese and yogurt, leafy green veggies, yellow or orange veggies like yellow squash, sweet potatoes, and carrots, as well as yellow-colored fruits. See, your color palette matters!

B-Complex

B-Complex vitamins are all involved with energy production, metabolism, and synthesis of hormones, as well as health of the nerves and function of the senses, so count on the Bs when you want more sexual pleasure. Also, for women, higher levels of B_5, pantothenic acid, and B_6, pyridoxine, can help balance the female hormones.

A deficiency of B_1, thiamine, will cause a lack of energy, inability to metabolize fats, proteins, and carbohydrates, and reduction in one's sex drive. A deficiency of B_3, niacin, can cause skin, bowel, and mental problems, as well as decreasing blood flow. So for men with high cholesterol and erectile dysfunction, more B_3 may help them overcome both because it assists in handling fats much the way statin drugs do, and it also increases blood flow through the body, thereby improving erectile function. Good foods that are high in B_1 include whole grains, nuts, beans, asparagus, and pineapple, while good sources of B_3 include lean meats, chicken, and fish, yogurt, peanuts, bran, and sun-dried tomatoes.

Vitamin C

Vitamin C, especially in large doses, is good at enhancing libido. So men with erectile dysfunction might improve their situation with three grams per day of vitamin C. Now, it should be noted that a study recommending this regimen used healthy and young volunteers, but the majority did increase their frequency of sexual intercourse. And again, it couldn't hurt to try it. In fact, vitamin C works wonders on the whole body, aiding in iron absorption for red blood cells and adrenal gland metabolism for hormone production, and both of these activities in turn improve energy production. This vitamin also strengthens the immune system, combats stress, and keeps the joints limber. We can recommend taking the powdered version, manufactured in Germany, rather than the pill version, manufactured in China, because the powder is much more rapidly usable by the body. And high doses should be broken up into three or four or five smaller doses, so the body gets its C-fix several times a day. Foods high in vitamin C include all citrus fruits like oranges and tangerines, strawberries and raspberries, dark leafy veggies, papayas and guavas, kiwis, broccoli and cauliflower, and peppers, especially chili peppers and all colors of bell peppers.

Vitamin D$_3$

Vitamin D$_3$ has been shown in studies to increase testosterone levels. And since vitamin D has for a very long time been known as "the sunshine vitamin," your doctor will probably tell you that the best way to get it is to spend at least 20 minutes a day out in the sunshine, soaking up rays, because the body will manufacture its own vitamin D as a result of sunshine hitting the skin. Of course, in winter when sunshine isn't readily available, you can take it in supplement form. It's also often added to milk and other drinks and is available through eating fish like wild salmon, tuna, or sole, taking fish oil, and eating pork, beef liver, or eggs, but just be sure you're getting enough of it all year round, as it also does other good things for the body besides making it sexy.

Vitamin E

Vitamin E is sometimes called the "sex vitamin" because it helps both genders produce sex hormones—which means it can improve a person's attraction, mood, and desire for sex. It's also an antioxidant, so it helps eliminate free radicals from the body and thereby helps keep the individual more youthful. And we've read lots of material lately suggesting it can actually be used as a lubricant during intercourse. Further, for men in particular, 400 mg of vitamin E can improve sperm motility, thereby increasing male fertility, especially when it's combined with 225 mcg of selenium. And with all the other healthy things vitamin E does, it also appears to boost libido—which would be a likely result of eliminating hormone imbalances. Good sources of vitamin E include nuts and seeds, especially sunflower seeds, pine nuts, safflower and cottonseed oil, peanuts, avocadoes, and tomatoes.

Vitamin K_2

Vitamin K_2 is another nutritional element that can help men have erections even into their elder years because K_2 is necessary for helping certain pathways close off during times of arousal. The highest amounts of the K vitamins are found in the dark, leafy green veggies like kale, collard greens, turnip greens, and spinach, but they're also plentiful in broccoli, herbs, the chili pepper family, asparagus, cabbage, and prunes.

DHEA

DHEA (dehydroepiandrosterone) is a hormone produced naturally by the adrenals, and it's primarily of concern for women, especially those who may be having a decrease in sexual interest as a result of decreases in production of the hormone because of age. Some people think it's a sort of Viagra for women, and because it's sold over the counter, it's an easy supplement to acquire. However, since it's a male hormone, women should check with their doctors to see if they need supplementation, as there's a slight risk of its causing breast cancer, heart attack, and excess hair growth in places women may not want it.

Arginine

Arginine is an amino acid, one of the many that make up a complete protein. This particular one is also considered a key to sexual arousal for both women and men because it increases the amount of blood flow through the sex organs, thus giving men longer-lasting erections and improving women's stimulation. Men can get results by taking it in pill form, while women may want to use it as a cream applied directly to where it's needed (yeah, the lady parts!) Arginine is found in meat, eggs, cheese, nuts, and coconut milk. In the body, it forms nitric oxide, which is the compound that increases genital blood flow.

Tyrosine

Tyrosine is another amino acid that's sometimes recommended for relieving stress and depression, both of which can inhibit sex drive in either gender. Of course, for getting a good supply of all the amino acids, be sure to eat plenty of protein daily.

Zinc

Zinc is an essential mineral for healthy sex organs because it's involved in the production of hormones. It's available in pill form, but there are lots of foods that can also provide it in high quantities, like practically all nuts and seeds, as well as oysters and dark chocolate, which are high on everybody's lists of aphrodisiac foods.

Part IV:
Fruits, Nuts, and Seeds

1. Fruits

Apricots

The English name of this delicious yellow-orange fruit was at one time "abrecock" or "apricock," and records show that in the court of King James I, "apricocks" were served as aphrodisiac sweets. Around this same time, William Shakespeare acknowledged apricots as having aphrodisiac powers in *A Midsummer Night's Dream.*

The Chinese cultivated apricots for more than 4,000 years, and Australian aboriginal people used them for aphrodisiac purposes, rubbing the genitals with the fruit's pulp as a perfume before sex. These luscious little fruits are a symbol of fertility in many cultures around the globe.

Apricots are high in potassium, magnesium, phosphorus, vitamins A and C, lycopene, and the anti-oxidant beta-carotene, and are a source of iron, necessary for female fertility.

Avocadoes

In ancient times, the Aztecs thought the dark green fruit of this plant hanging in pairs from the tree looked like human testicles, so they called the tree *ahuacuatl,* which translates as "testicle tree." And one has to admit that the fruit of this plant is voluptuous, from its sexy-looking outside to its smooth, creamy insides. The early Spanish church fathers apparently thought so, too, as they banned the eating of them. But avocadoes are rich in all kinds of nutrients that contribute not just to testosterone production but also to lowering cholesterol, healing the liver, and fighting cancer, and their minerals, vitamins, and especially folic acid are important for females as well. So everybody will benefit from nibbling the fruit of the "testicle tree." Guacamole, anyone?

Bananas

The banana is another example of a fruit once believed through sympathetic magic to bring on sexual prowess because of its marvelous phallic shape. But as the #1 item sold through Walmart, this plant's popularity may also be attributed to its taste and not just its aphrodisiac reputation.

Nutritionally, bananas contain B vitamins, magnesium, and potassium, necessary for the production of sex hormones, especially testosterone, and for raising the body's energy levels They also contain bromelain, an enzyme that increases male libido.

A myth from Islamic culture says that after Eve gave Adam the apple from the Tree of Knowledge and they realized they were naked, they didn't cover their privates with the leaves of figs but rather with banana leaves. So for Muslims, there's a very sexy connection with bananas to what is generally thought to have been the first sexual experience of our first parents.

Cherries

The most obvious association of sex with cherries is the English slang word for the female hymen, although the name of this fruit actually derives from the French word "cerise," which is the term for its color.

Historically, cherries have been prescribed as both aphrodisiac and analgesic remedies, the latter specifically used for relieving the pain of gout and arthritis. These luscious little fruits are loaded with A, C, and E, are high in the potassium needed by the body for hormone and pheromone production, plus magnesium, folic acid, iron, and antioxidants to keep you healthy and youthful. And they're just terrific dipped in chocolate, another food with a long reputation as a an aphrodisiac.

Date Palm

The date palm's fruit is a date, which is said to be the "Sacred Fruit of the Arabs." Of course, the Jews also ate dates and fermented them into wine. Among the Jews, dates were considered a symbol for elegance and grace, and they were often given as gifts to women. The Jewish word for date was "tamar," which is the name King David bestowed on his beautiful daughter, Tamar.

Dates probably go back to prehistoric times, for they were mentioned in the records of the first historic civilizations and were cultivated as far back as ancient Mesopotamia and Egypt, though they spread eventually to the sunnier climes of Asia, northern Africa, Italy, and Spain; the Spanish brought them to Mexico and California.

Figs

The inside of a fig is thought by some to resemble the female genitalia, so figs have traditionally been considered a sexual stimulant. When a male breaks open a fig and eats it while his lover is watching, it could certainly be perceived as an erotic invitation.

In a great deal of religious art, Adam and Eve are shown in the Garden of Eden wearing fig leaves after their fall, so the fig symbolizes both their sexuality (the ripe fruit with its female sexual connection) and the modesty the first couple demonstrated by using the fig leaves to cover their nakedness. In fact, some Old Testament experts believe the fig, rather than the apple, was the fruit hanging on the Tree of Knowledge in Eden.

Figs are known to contain high amounts of amino acids, which increase libido and sexual stamina. They're also high in flavonoids, potassium, antioxidants, and polyphenols, so they're good for maintaining health and youth.

Figs symbolized fertility and love among the ancient Greeks, who considered them a sacred food. And they were the favorite fruit of Queen Cleopatra of Egypt, who was never a slacker in pursuit of sexual gratification.

Goji Berries

Goji berries belong to the family of nightshades and thus are relatives of the tomato, the potato, eggplants, chili peppers and capsicum plants, gooseberries, belladonna, mandrake, and tobacco.

Known in China as "happy berries," these nutritious little fruits are touted for their aphrodisiac powers. Believed to increase testosterone levels, research has shown their efficacy in the treatment of metabolic syndrome, which often precedes erectile dysfunction. They have recently made a splash in the West as the basis for a nutrition juice, although the Chinese use them as a source for fruit wine.

Grapes

The history of these sweet finger foods can be traced back to ancient Egypt, which seems to have been the first culture to turn them into wine. In ancient Greece, they were sacred to the god Dionysus, known as Bacchus among the Romans, and in both these cultures, they were symbols of love, fertility, and virility, as well as of sexual ecstasy, which was also governed by this god. In Greece, newlyweds were given clusters of grapes in the belief that the seeds would bring them children.

High in vitamins A and C, potassium, and antioxidants, grapes are both a sweet and a healthy love treat before sex. And frozen grapes are also a delicious way to cool drinks in summer—especially the wine you might share with a lover.

Mangoes

Shaped like avocadoes, mangoes can be used as an alternate to those luscious fruits, offering similar benefits in terms of stimulating the mind to think of testicles. In fact, in many cultures, like Thailand, mangoes were considered symbols of male sexuality, and in India men were even prescribed "mango therapy" to improve their sexual performance.

Olives and Olive Oil

The Greeks believed that eating olives made men more virile. But the fact is, pure virgin olive oil and the olives from which it comes are super-high in antioxidants and a terrific source of monounsaturated and polyunsaturated fats, necessary for heart and circulation health and production of hormones, all of which contribute to a better sex life.

Papaya

In the Philippines, the papaya is used to *control* libido, but in Guatemala, it's considered an aphrodisiac. Nothing quite explains this paradox, unless maybe it's a libido control for one gender but an aphrodisiac for the other.

Papaya is estrogenic, which means it has compounds that act in the body the same way as does the female hormone estrogen, although some authorities say this is true only of green, unripe papaya. Papaya has been used in folk medicine for centuries to promote healthy menstruation and milk production, as well as to improve the female libido and facilitate childbirth. It is also high in antioxidants like folic acid and vitamins A, C, and E, which promote healthy hormone production in both genders.

Maybe guys should get a slightly larger share of the avocado appetizers, and the ladies can have a bigger portion of the papaya dessert.

Pomegranates

The pomegranate is a pretty red fruit that looks a lot like an apple, but inside it has sweet, plump, fruity seeds surrounded by a pulp, which, though it can be pretty, can also be quite bitter.

In ancient Greece, seeds of the pomegranate were offered to Ceres, goddess of grain, known in ancient Rome as Demeter, because of the belief that they brought fertility. Persephone, called Proserpina in Rome, was Ceres' daughter, who was carried off by Hades, known in Rome as Pluto, god of the underworld. Ceres went looking for her daughter to bring her home, but she found her moments after the girl had eaten six seeds of a pomegranate. For her mistake of eating the six seeds, Persephone was required to stay in the underworld for six months of the year through the fall and winter. The other six months she could spend back in her mother's company during the grain-growing season on the surface of the planet. Perhaps because of this association with Persephone, the pomegranate was also known among the Greeks as the "fruit of the dead."

The pomegranate was used in later Christian culture in paintings of both Mary Magdalene and the Virgin Mary and on the Tarot card of the High Priestess, where palm leaves and pomegranates form the shape of the Tree of Life, so it may have been associated with sexuality, like Eve's apple, or it may have had a much deeper symbolic meaning. Some Jewish scholars believe the pomegranate was in fact the real fruit Eve ate and offered to Adam in the Garden of Eden.

The clearest aphrodisiac association for this pretty red fruit, however, is with its high content of polyphenols, with large amounts of vitamins C and K, and with its ancient name, *"panspermia,"* suggesting it might have the effect of increasing the male sperm count.

And a recent study indicated that pomegranate juice has an effect in erasing erectile dysfunction. Possibly because they are high in tannins, in ancient India parts of the pomegranate were inserted into the vagina because they were considered to have both contraceptive and abortifacient powers. We, however, have found no actual evidence of the efficacy of this early "morning after" pill.

Pineapple

Pineapple is a purifier and a diuretic, and like papaya, it has a positive effect on digestion. It has also been used historically in the homeopathic cure for impotence. If it actually works, it's probably because it's very high in vitamin C, essential for healthy hormone production. It also contains loads of antioxidants, supporting youth and vibrancy, and is a rich source of manganese, which is necessary for sexual health, so that's probably where it gets its aphrodisiac reputation.

Raspberries and Strawberries

Sometimes described as "fruit nipples," raspberries and strawberries are full of vitamin C and have the reputation for increasing libido. These are friendly foods to feed a lover while listening to sexy music or even just thinking sexy thoughts. Strawberries in particular were considered the love fruits of the Roman goddess of love, Venus, perhaps because of their red color and heart-like shape. In France, they were once fed to newlyweds as a cold soup in order to prepare them sexually for their honeymoon.

Some people enhance the sweetness of these sexual treasures by dipping them in chocolate, honey, or powdered sugar before hand-feeding them to a lover. (Umm, this description is beginning to *feel* like a Roman banquet—"Feed me a strawberry, Julius, and let's see where it leads.")

Saw Palmetto

This plant is a small, 3-6 foot-high palm, which can live to be more than 500 years old.

It has the reputation for improving circulation in the genitals, and its fruits can be eaten or its juice fermented into a love drink. It contains fatty acids, essential oils, and phytosterols. In traditional herbal medicine, the Mayans used saw palmetto as a tonic, and the Seminoles used the berries as an antiseptic and expectorant. Other American Indians used it to treat urinary tract and reproductive system problems, and these uses seem to be where it got its reputation as an aphrodisiac.

Today, saw palmetto extract is a popular treatment for benign prostatic hyperplasia, which is commonly found in older men.

Watermelon

Watermelon contains lycopene and beta-carotene, which are both cancer-fighting nutrients and good enough reasons to enjoy this super juicy summer treat. But in addition, a recent study shows that the rind of watermelon has large amounts of the amino acid *citrulline*, which is a key intermediate in the urea cycle, by which humans excrete ammonia. And citrulline is also known to be beneficial for the immune function. Further, citrulline triggers the amino acid *arginine* to function, and this is the Viagra chemical that revs up the cardiovascular system, getting blood pumped up and ready to go where it's needed. So while eating watermelon isn't likely to give someone the same effect as taking Viagra, maybe eating pickled watermelon rind will get closer to it.

2. Nuts

A nut in the kitchen isn't necessarily the same as a nut in the botanist's boudoir. Take a shell, put a large and somewhat oily kernel in it, and a cook will call it a nut. The botanist will tell you that a nut has a *very* hard shell, and the seed remains attached to the ovary wall, making it a lot harder to extract than most of those fruits we generally call nuts.

But even a botanist might not make the distinction in the kitchen between *true* nuts, such as walnuts, pecans, chestnuts, and hazelnuts, and what are termed *culinary* nuts, such as almonds, brazil nuts, cashews, macadamias, and pistachios.

Heck, a cook will even call a peanut—which is a legume—or a pine nut—which is a seed—a nut. What a nut!

Almonds

All nuts are high in zinc, contain essential fatty acids, support the libido, and assist with the production of hormones. But almonds in particular have had a connection with human sexuality for centuries. A symbol of fertility throughout the ages, almonds have an aroma that supposedly is a turn-on for women, which may be why they're used in many women's soaps and beauty products—indeed, Honora remembers as a child thinking that Jergen's lotion, which her mother especially liked for her hands, smelled like almonds.

Almonds are high in magnesium and vitamin E, both of which do enhance fertility and support the libido. The French author Alexander Dumas supposedly had almond soup every night in order to be prepared for lovemaking, and Samson is said to have wooed Delilah with almond branches.

Cashews

These yummy nuts are considered to have aphrodisiac properties in Brazil, where they are consumed for libido enhancement as well as other medicinal purposes, such as lowering blood pressure and reducing fever.

3. Seeds

Without going into considerable detail concerning the biological definition of a seed, and then trying to explain why we've made the kinds of divisions and distinctions that we've used in this little book, let us just consider a seed to be that part of a flowering plant that can be sown in order to produce a new plant.

Or it can be eaten as an aphrodisiac—as you wish.

Anise Seed

Anise, or aniseed, is a flowering plant found in southwest Asia and the eastern Mediterranean.

Anise has long been popular as an aphrodisiac, going back to Greek and Roman times, where the seeds were sucked as a means of getting turned on. It has a taste similar to licorice (so for those who don't like that flavor, you can move on to the next item in this list). Because it contains estrogen-like compounds, anise has been prescribed in herbal medicine for menstrual cramps. It's also popular as a cooking spice on practically every continent (except Antarctica, where the native population of penguins don't do much cooking), and in India it's used as a digestive after meals, perhaps because it's also said to decrease flatulence.

Pumpkin Seeds

Pumpkin seeds are high in magnesium, zinc, and omega 3 fatty acids. Zinc contributes to the health of the sex organs, while the omega 3 fatty acids promote production of prostaglandins. And magnesium increases the production of testosterone. So what can grow from a little pumpkin seed? Guess!

Pine Nuts

Pine nuts are actually seeds. All pines have seeds that are edible, but only about 20 of them have seeds large enough to be considered as a crop.

The second century Roman physician and scholar Galen of Pergamon recommended eating a hundred pine nuts before going to bed, so perhaps modern bodybuilders who chomp on pine nuts to help increase their stamina actually know something the rest of us don't.

These little gems from the evergreen pine are high in zinc content, a key mineral in male potency maintenance and essential for testosterone production. Used during the Middle Ages in love potions in Europe and sprinkled in the beds of lovers in Arabia to stimulate the libido, pine nuts have been found to increase cardiovascular function, always necessary to help get the blood flowing to one's extremities, including the private ones.

Sunflowers and Sunflower Seeds

Sunflower petals made into a tea have long been believed to create a sexually stimulating result. They contain vitamin E and chlorogenic acid, both of which are supposed to have a powerful effect on sexual desire. Sunflower seeds are high in zinc, which is stimulating to the sex organs. Maybe you could get the best of both parts of the plant by putting the leaves in a salad and sprinkling the seeds on top.

Part V: Vegetables

1. Flower Buds

Artichoke

Full of vitamins K, C, folic acid, and antioxidants, artichokes are reputed to assist blood flow, and we know how important that is for the pleasurable sex experiences of both genders. According to Greek mythology, the god Zeus (who had an unbelievably varied history of adventures with the fair sex) is supposed to have created the artichoke when he turned one of his would-be lovers into this prickly-looking veggie because she spurned his advances. However, herbal doctors through the ages have used it as an aphrodisiac, as well as a breath freshener, deodorant, and diuretic.

In the 16th century, it is claimed that only males were allowed to eat artichokes because of their effects on sexual arousal (they didn't want women getting aroused and sexually uncontrollable). In fact, Catherine de Medici scandalized the French court by eating large numbers of artichokes—but then she was Italian before she became the Queen of France, so what did she care about what people thought?

It appears Catherine's preference for artichokes later caught on among the French, for street vendors in Paris in the 18th century touted the sexually-arousing effects of artichokes as a selling point.

Broccoli

This green giant of a healthy veggie is reputed to be an aphrodisiac for men because it increases testosterone production and boosts libido through a compound called indole-3-carbinol, but for the same reason, it's not so great as an aphrodisiac for women because it inhibits estrogen production. Nevertheless, if getting sexy isn't the goal, then broccoli is a terrific side dish, because it's cancer inhibiting and full of vitamins. Otherwise, just the guys should eat it right before sex.

2. Leaves

Lovage

This plant can be used in a similar way to parsley, and in fact, its name comes from "love-ache," because "ache" was a medieval name for parsley. In the Middle Ages, witches used lovage in love potions, a fact that may be the source of its reputation as an aphrodisiac. However, it also tastes and smells very much like celery, which can be a turn-on for women. It's native to southern European countries and popular there simply for its culinary uses, wherein its leaves can be used as an herb or in salads, its roots can be chopped in salads or cooked into soups, and its seeds are often added to dishes as a spice.

However, lovage should not be eaten by pregnant women because of possible abortifacient results or by those who have kidney disease.

Spinach

Do you really want to know why Popeye "fights to the finitch" when he eats his spinach? It's because this dark green veggie contains large amounts of arginine, which the body needs to produce nitric oxide and improve blood flow. It's also very high in vitamins A, K, D, E, and trace minerals, plus omega-3 fatty acids, protects the body against cancer, turns the body more alkaline, is good for the eyes, and gives you stronger bones. So guys, eat your spinach for better erections, and get all kinds of other health benefits, too.

3. Stems

Asparagus

Ancient Greeks and Arabs cultivated asparagus because of its supposed aphrodisiac properties. As a result of the "sympathetic magic" associated with its phallic shape, asparagus is one of those foods eaten as an aphrodisiac because its shape may similarly shape up your sex life. It's said that people who eat large amounts of asparagus generally have lots of lovers, though its shape would suggest this applies primarily to men; one story says that French bridegrooms in the 19th century would eat three servings of asparagus as a prenuptial meal. However, the 17th century English herbalist Nicholas Culpeper believed it would stir up lust in both men and women. Asparagus is rich in vitamin E, which stimulates testosterone production. However, because it's also full of vitamins A, B, and C, and especially folic acid, it could certainly assist both sexes in increasing libido and attaining orgasm.

There is another side effect however—that strangely pungent yet sweet urine odor that can often be detected as soon as 15 to 30 minutes after eating asparagus. And if you think that *you* don't produce this particular odor because you can't smell it in your own urine, then it's your olfactory genes that are at play, not any special digestive secret you may have!

Susan's mother used to quote a sign posted in a club in London: "Gentlemen will please refrain from urinating in the umbrella stand during asparagus season."

Celery

Again we're looking at a vegetable that probably got its reputation as an aphrodisiac because its head (the stalks and leaves) is incredibly phallic, but in addition it has lots of minerals, including calcium and magnesium, iron, phosphorus, and sulfur. It's been used since the Middle Ages as a cure for impotence and a strengthener of the sex organs, possibly because it also contains androstenone, which is a male pheromone. Maybe the bottom line is that if a guy eats enough celery, he'll smell like celery and thereby attract women.

4. Rhizomes and Tubers

A rhizome is an underground plant stem with nodes that can store starches, proteins, and nutrients for the plant, and send out new roots and stems, creating a new plant.

If a part of a rhizome is enlarged for storage, particularly of starches, we have a tuber.

Ginger

Acknowledged in the *Kama Sutra* of India as a turn-on, ginger is hot stuff whether eaten in food or made into a tea. It stimulates circulation of the blood by raising the heart rate, thereby increasing the flow of blood to the sex organs. And its pleasant scent and health benefits are good for both genders.

Potatoes, Sweet Potatoes, and Yams

While only distantly related, all three of these are tubers. Potatoes are in the Nightshade family, sweet potatoes are in the Morning Glory family, and a yam is a yam is a yam.

In Shakespeare's day, potatoes were considered to be an aphrodisiac, as suggested by his use of them in *The Merry Wives of Windsor* along with a couple of other sweetmeats with sexual connotations and a reference to the song "Green Sleeves." Indeed, one authority suggests that both white and sweet potatoes were considered aphrodisiac foods when they were first introduced to European cuisine from the Americas because they were rare and considered a delicacy.

Said to be particularly stimulating for a woman's sex drive, the sweet potato is high in potassium, good for reducing stress, and also high in vitamin C, calcium, folic acid, and beta-carotene, the antioxidant that the body converts to vitamin A. In fact, sweet potatoes are so high in nutrients that the Center for Science in the Public Interest has rated them the most nutritious veggie. With all these positives going for them, there's no wonder sweet potatoes are recommended as a superlatively sexy side dish before a night of love!

Wild yam has been recommended for years as an assist to gynecological problems, and it turns out it contains the chemical diosgenin, which is similar to female sex hormones. So some doctors actually recommend that wild yam cream be massaged into the genitals of women heading toward menopause who find they aren't producing enough vaginal fluids to make sex comfortable.

5. Roots

Beets

The French word for beet, *betterave*, is also a slang word for the penis. Because of their high boron content, beets have been favored to increase virility and sexual prowess in males since the time of the Romans, but they're actually also responsible for increasing sex hormones in women. This may be true, because prostitutes were supposedly told in the early 20th century that they could, "Take favors in the beetroot fields."

Beets are good for building the blood and are rich in several of the B-complex vitamins, plus A and C, magnesium, potassium, calcium, phosphorus, and iron. In addition, they balance the body's pH from acidity to alkalinity, help cleanse the liver, gall bladder, kidneys, and bladder, balance blood sugar levels, and help normalize brain function. Good for your love life and your health, beets really can't be beat!

Carrots

According to a Japanese proverb, "A man who likes carrots likes women." The phallic carrot is yet another veggie that may excite simply by its shape. Carrots are good for the eyes because they contain loads of vitamins and beta-carotene. Are they also good for the sex organs? Well, Middle Eastern royals thought so in the past, as they reputedly used these orange pleasure sticks as instruments of seduction—hm-m-m, we wonder how?

Ginseng

The Chinese have been using ginseng as an aphrodisiac for thousands of years to treat men with low sex drive and erectile dysfunction, especially when they are the result of stress and fatigue. Like many of the other plant-based stimulants described here, ginseng has properties that increase blood flow to the genital area, increase sex-related hormones, and enhance sexual appetite as well as sexual response.

In addition to helping men through erectile dysfunction problems, ginseng also seems to help women increase desire and boost performance, energy, and orgasm. Over half of all men and women in studies using ginseng reported being in the mood more often. However, because of its estrogen-producing effects, ginseng isn't recommended for pregnant or nursing women. Its only other reported effect is that it produces excitability, so it's wise to have one's partner handy when having a nice cup of ginseng tea.

Maca

Maca is a form of ginseng that grows in Peruvian high-altitude areas. The ancient Incas used it to give their warriors extra strength in battle, but its most legendary ability lies in improving lust and giving both men and women better orgasms. And modern research on both animals and humans shows it does increase libido and stamina, though it seems to work best on men (and male lab rats).

Most commonly available in the U.S. in supplement form, maca roots contain high amounts of minerals, such as calcium, magnesium, iron, and selenium, as well as amino acids, fatty acids, and aromatic isothiocyanates that are said to have aphrodisiac properties. And should you encounter it in its natural plant form, it tastes like nuts, in case that's a plus for you.

6. Bulbs

Onions

Like garlic, their vegetable drawer companion, onions have the reputation as an aphrodisiac because they heat the body. They were forbidden to be eaten by Tibetan priests and monks, for it was feared they would stir up their passions. Onions were mentioned in both Arabic and Indian texts as contributive to the art of love making, and in old France, onion soup was traditionally served to newlyweds the day after their first night together to restore their sexual desire.

Garlic

Eating garlic creates heat, which is said to stir sexual desires. Remember the Pardoner in Chaucer's *Canterbury Tales*, who smelled of garlic, onions, and leeks? That was included to give the reader a clue to the character's sexual predispositions.

Garlic is used in much Italian and French cooking, but with the understanding that "everybody eats some," so when you're indulging in it, be sure you share it with your partner. Garlic has been used for centuries to cure everything from the common cold to heart ailments, and the truth is, its essential oils have antibiotic properties. Further, it's been used as an aphrodisiac since the time of the ancient Egyptians, and the Romans later dedicated it to Ceres, their goddess of fertility. In ancient Tibet, monks weren't allowed to enter their monasteries if they'd been eating garlic because, as with onions, it was reputed to stir up the passions.

The truth is that the lowly garlic is extremely high in arginine, which stimulates the body's production of nitric oxide for blood vessel dilation. Garlic also contains allicin, which helps get the blood flowing to the sexual organs.

Garlic is actually a blood thinner, so it's always puzzled us as to why it would banish vampires, since they *need* blood to be thin so they can drink it. Oh, well, that's just the magic of garlic!

Shallots

The shallot is a variety of onion that grows into multiple bulbs from a single bulb, so it looks a bit like a bulb of garlic. It is sweeter, milder, more aromatic, and has a richer flavor and a firmer texture than other varieties of onion. It's also more expensive, but a fancy gourmet meal cooked in your own kitchen and served up to someone special can be a turn-on for both of you.

7. Fruits Used as Vegetables

Cucumber

If we're talking about the sympathetic magic of the similar shapes of things, I'll bet one of the first images that comes to mind regarding the shape of the male sex organ is the cucumber. However, a recent study by the Smell and Taste Treatment and Research Foundation in Chicago demonstrated that the smell of cucumbers and female arousal are directly related.

Also, cucumber contains vitamin C and manganese, both of which are on the list of nutrients for maintaining sexual health, as well as silica, which supports connective tissues and keeps us youthful and supple. So don't judge a cuke by just its (sexy) shape.

Okra

Okra is a stiff vegetable and has a sort of slimy fluid. Now, doesn't that make you think of sex? Well, it should, because okra also has lots of magnesium and hence is naturally relaxing. Plus it has iron, zinc, vitamin B, and folic acid to assist with healthy sex organs and vitality. Could this be why the Cajun French in Louisiana eat so much gumbo?

Squash

Many types of squash around the planet are considered to be aphrodisiacs, some perhaps because of their lovely penis shape, and some because they are high in nutritional content that may, in fact, contribute to better health generally and better sexual health specifically. The seeds of many species are full of fatty oil, protein, and vitamin E; in Ayurvedic medicine, some types of squash seeds are eaten during love rituals and to assist in healing male impotence. Other cultures view the squash seeds as aphrodisiacs for women. But don't just eat the seeds and leave the rest behind, as all forms of this veggie make for healthy eating.

Tomatoes

The first tomatoes brought from South America to Europe were shunned because they were believed to be either poisonous or immoral. Into the 1800s, members of some religious groups linked the tomato to Eve's apple and referred to it as another "forbidden fruit," fearing its slutty scarlet color and smooth, sexy skin might fill young members of the congregation with lust. However, both France and Italy shortly came to realize what they were missing and labeled this tangy, sweet, and succulent delight the "love apple" (*pomme d'amour* in French and *poma amoris* in Italian) perhaps because of its presumed aphrodisiac powers.

Tomatoes are members of the nightshade family, related to belladonna, which may explain why they were originally considered toxic and also why they came to be viewed as aphrodisiacs. But it takes far less belladonna to poison a potential partner than it does to do the same deed with tomatoes.

Part VI:
Herbs

Some green plants just cry out to have their leaves used fresh as a garnish on a fancy dinner plate or dried and crushed and stirred into a soup or stew as a seasoning. These are herbs. (Spices we'll look at in the next section.)

1. Parsley, Sage, Rosemary, and Thyme

When these herbs are listed in a group, most of us burst into a chorus of *Scarborough Fair*, the strange song by a lover who sets impossible tasks for the woman who once was his true love. All these herbs are still currently used in cooking. But what did these tasty little food additives really mean in the song? Let's look at some of their properties before we hazard a guess.

Parsley

Omigosh! That innocent looking little sprig of pretty green garnish on your plate is reputed to have aphrodisiac sex-stimulating powers, and to have been not only an ingredient of love potions in the past but also an additive mixed into witches' flying ointments. It's also claimed to be an irritant that in high doses can cause an abortion.

Who knew (besides the witches, of course)?

But wait just a darn minute, please—if it's so sexy, scary, and psychotropic, how come the Greek physician Hippocrates recommended it highly as a treatment for urinary tract problems? The answer is that it's a natural diuretic, which helps to flush toxins from the body by increasing urine output. It's also loaded with nutrients that contribute to the health of the sex organs, like vitamins A, B_1, and B_6. A cup of minced parsley has more vitamin C than two oranges, more beta-carotene than a big carrot, as much calcium as a glass of milk, and 20 times the iron of a piece of liver. And not only that, but

39

chewing a sprig of parsley freshens the breath, and it's supposed to be good also for improving digestion. Medieval herbalists prescribed it for taking away bitterness, both in the physical and the spiritual sense.

However, because parsley contains a high amount of oxalates, we have read warnings that pregnant or nursing women should check with their doctors before consuming large amounts of parsley, taking parsley powder, or drinking infusions containing parsley because of its possible abortifacient properties. Forewarned is forearmed.

And so far as its reputation for being psychotropic goes, we couldn't find any warnings about how it might cause you to fly around at night on a broom—or at least think that's what you're doing.

So if you're not pregnant, go ahead, eat that sprig of garnish on your plate—maybe its breath-freshening capability is what really makes it an aphrodisiac.

Sage

Common sage (*salvia officinalis*) has the reputation for symbolizing strength, and it's an especially tasty additive to dishes that include chicken, turkey, and other kinds of fowl. It's also considered by some authorities to be a uterine stimulant. But clary sage (*salvia sclarea*) for hundreds of years was considered a woman's botanical, and even today the essential oil of this plant is often used in a bath or a massage for getting through a menstrual cycle with ease because of its calming and mood-balancing influence, while it's antispasmodic and sedative properties are purported to ease menstrual cramps. It's also reputed to be a sexual stimulant for women.

In medieval times, sage was considered both a contraceptive and an abortifacient, so like parsley, it's not to be used by pregnant women.

Rosemary

The most famous quote associated with rosemary is in Shakespeare's *Hamlet*, when Ophelia hands the prince a sprig of evergreen, saying, "There's rosemary—that's for remembrance." Rosemary has long been associated with fidelity in love, so Ophelia is reminding Hamlet they had been lovers, and she wants him to remember their love. In England, it has been a tradition for brides to wear sprigs of rosemary in their hair on their wedding day.

Rosemary is another herb with an aphrodisiac reputation, reputedly working both on the skin in a bath or a massage oil or when ingested, for it contains an essential oil that can have psychotropic effects if taken in large amounts. But don't do that if you're pregnant because, like parsley and sage, rosemary in high doses can be an abortifacient.

Rosemary also contains nutrients that assist with circulation of the blood, and it's one of the few plants in which its nutrients become more accessible after its leaves are dried. But perhaps its aphrodisiac reputation is because of its strong scent, which increases mental alertness and strengthens memory. And ladies need to know that as the scent of celery and cucumber arouse sexual interest in women, so the smell of rosemary arouses sexual desire in men.

Rosemary was associated in ancient times with the goddess Aphrodite/Venus, who can sometimes be seen in iconography wearing or holding a sprig of it, and this is yet another explanation as to why it's considered an aphrodisiac.

Thyme

Thyme has traditionally symbolized courage, but this may be courage for women since this plant is associated with feminine love. It, too, is a women's botanical, acting as a uterine stimulant, an aid to better menstrual blood flow, and easy periods. But like parsley, sage, and rosemary, it's not recommended for pregnant women because of its possible abortifacient properties.

A legend associated with thyme is that at Midsummer, also known as Summer Solstice, the King of the Fairies makes an appearance in order to dance in a field of wild thyme. Though this sounds like something out of Shakespeare's *A Midsummer Night's Dream*, this seems a significant association with thyme's aphrodisiac reputation since Midsummer in European countries is traditionally a celebration of the fecundity of the earth and of human sexuality. The sexy season starts at Beltane, May 1st, which begins the lustiest month of the year, and runs to Teltane, August 1st, when the spring crops have reached harvest time. And the midpoint of that season is Summer Solstice, so it's often celebrated with great sexual enthusiasm.

So what's going on in the song "Scarborough Fair"? The lover asks to be remembered to "one who lives there" who was once his true love. Why is she no longer a true love, and why does he set her some seemingly impossible tasks? If we look at the herbs listed in the song, we can see they all seem to affect women, working as aphrodisiacs, contraceptives, and abortifacients. So sex is definitely involved in the song's meaning. Was the woman knowledgeable about the properties of the herbs? Did she use them to protect against or interrupt a pregnancy? Is the lover suggesting by the tasks he sets that she has some knowledge of magic or witchcraft? Maybe all of the above—or maybe after all it's just a sweet, sad song about unrequited love.

2. Other Herbs (Besides the Ones at Scarborough Fair)

Arugula

The ancient Romans dedicated this spicy herb and current salad veggie to their sex god Priapus and are said to have used it in love potions—and probably with good nutritional reason, since it's packed with all the vitamins, minerals, and phytochemicals most needed for healthy sexual functioning. It is also said to protect against cancer and macular degeneration, boost the immune system, and detox the body, and presumably these added attractions are all going on while you're having a good time in the bedroom.

Dill

Dill has been a popular herb since 3000 BCE, where in the Mediterranean area it was prized for its medicinal uses. Used in ancient Assyria, Egypt, Greece, Rome, and Europe for improving digestion and soothing stomach ailments, it was also believed to have magical properties and was used in love potions and as an aphrodisiac. Because it was thought to enhance endurance, women would add it to their lovers' wine to increase their sexual staying power and passion.

Perhaps because of its association with magic, dill was hung in sprigs around the home during the Middle Ages in order to protect against evil or witchcraft. Along these same lines, in some European countries, dill was believed to bring good fortune and happiness, so brides would wear or carry sprigs of dill on their wedding day to bring luck and joy in marriage.

Ayurvedic medicine has used dill in at least 56 medical treatments. It's known to function as a protector against free-radicals and carcinogens, has anti-bacterial properties, and is high in calcium, magnesium, iron, and manganese. So aren't you glad to know about all these interesting associations for dill? It's not just for pickles after all!

Mint

The name of this herbal plant derives from the Greek myth of Minthe, a nymph who was dazzled by Hades in his chariot and was on the verge of seducing him when his wife, Persephone, turned her into the mint plant. Mint was also used in Greece in the entheogenic drink of fermented barley that was given to participants in the Eleusinian mysteries, which offered hope for life after death. However, Aristotle is said to have advised Alexander the Great not to let his men drink mint tea before a battle because it was an aphrodisiac and would take their minds away from fighting.

Sarsaparilla

Native to Mexico and the tropical forests of Central and South America and the Caribbean, sarsaparilla is an herb that has been used for centuries in the treatment of hormonal conditions that cause libido loss in both men and women, as well as male impotence and a whole raft of other sexual disorders. It is also believed that sarsaparilla may help to keep the glandular system in balance.

In traditional Chinese medicine and in South American shamanic treatments, sarsaparilla was used to treat leprosy, while in Indian medicine, it was a treatment for snakebite, perhaps because it seemed to have anti-venom properties.

Because it is both anti-inflammatory and anti-bacterial, it has also been administered as a blood toner and remedy for inflammatory diseases, and to treat skin disorders like psoriasis and venereal diseases such as syphilis and gonorrhea. More than one source has suggested that in the Wild West, men would stop by the local bar and have a drink of sarsaparilla before going to the local brothels as a way of protecting themselves from these social diseases.

Sarsaparilla contains vitamins A, C, D, and B-complex, as well as calcium, iron, chromium, copper, cobalt, zinc, magnesium, manganese, phosphorus, tin, potassium, silicon, sodium, sulfur, iodine and the amino acids cysteine and methionine.

Sarsaparilla contains the steroid saponin diosgenin, an essential component of the steroid hormones testosterone, estrogen, and progesterone. Diosgenin is the substance that was used to create the first birth control pills in the 1960s, so it has been suggested sarsaparilla may produce estrogen-like effects in the body. However, women who are undergoing treatment for hormone-driven cancer or who are on oral birth control should not take sarsaparilla root, nor should women who are pregnant or breastfeeding, as the effect of the hormonal elements of the plant on fetuses and nursing infants are not known.

Sarsaparilla may cause an allergic reaction in some people. It may irritate the stomach lining or increase urine production and thereby irritate the kidneys. It is not recommended for people who have kidney disease. It is also not recommended for people who are on blood thinners or prostate medications. And because it can increase absorption of such chemicals as digitalis or bismuth, those taking sarsaparilla should avoid use of these elements during that time.

Yarrow

Yarrow is also a powerful healing herb, containing natural painkillers like salicylic acid, and has been used for centuries for staunching the blood flow of wounds. In Homer's *Iliad*, the centaur Chiron taught Achilles the properties of yarrow so he could heal the wounded Greek soldiers in the Trojan War. Hence, it is also useful in the treatment of menstrual problems. An essential oil made from yarrow can be used as an anti-inflammatory.

It is said that the Navaho tribes used yarrow as an aphrodisiac to enhance performance, ingesting it an hour or two before intercourse either in a tea or by chewing the raw stem. In the 1600s its leaves were a popular vegetable, while both its leaves and flowers have been used in the making of certain liquors.

Part VII:
Spices

What exactly is a spice? Take any part of a plant that you want—usually (but not always) seeds, fruits, roots, or bark—dry it, and use it for flavoring, coloring, or food preservation. That's a spice.

Basil

A favorite spice in Europe and South Asia, basil also is supposed to have a positive effect on one's sex life by increasing both sex drive and fertility. Its aroma would fit with the idea that perfumes can function as aphrodisiacs—indeed, women once dusted their breasts with dried basil so men would want to kiss them—but sweet basil also tastes really good, especially in Italian pasta sauces. Full of vitamins, basil also has the reputation for increasing blood circulation, and we know by now which body parts this can be good for!

Black Peppercorns

Black pepper is one of the five spices mentioned in the *Kama Sutra* as being aphrodisiac. One of the world's oldest spice crops, it is native to the southern part of India. It was so highly prized in the Middle Ages that it was often used as currency, and desire for its increased availability encouraged the explorers of the Age of Exploration to find new routes to the Far East.

Today, peppercorns, whether black, white, or green, are used worldwide more than any other spice, with over 60,000 tons consumed annually.

Like all other peppers, black pepper heats the blood, thereby increasing blood flow to the genitals, which may be why it was prescribed in early times for impotency. It does have anti-bacterial properties and is a good source of vitamins C and K, potassium, manganese, iron, and potassium. It's also a good anti-inflammatory, an anti-oxidant, and good for treating digestive problems, respiratory disorders, anemia, skin and muscle problems, and dental issues, and it even assists in weight loss. So sprinkle a little on whatever you like— and just see where it leads!

Cardamom

Both green and black cardamom are used as flavorings, cooking spices and medicines, but green cardamom is considered the true spice. Ground cardamom costs $6 to $10 per ounce—among the spices only saffron and vanilla cost more, so this is indeed a rich treat! Once the seed is ground, it can quickly lose its flavor, so the pod is often ground with the seed to lower the price, and of course the quality.

This spice can be a stimulant for the body, reputed to cool it when it's hot and warm it when it's cold, so add it to coffee, either iced or hot, for an added seasonal pleasure. It's often used as an essential oil in massage because of its erotic effect. Here's a clue as to its powers: Cleopatra is supposed to have used it in her baths. But it's also great for eating as a culinary spice.

Cayenne and Other Hot Chili Peppers

Cayenne and other chili peppers, like pepperoncini and paprika, are high in vitamin C and are yet more plants that assist blood circulation, increasing blood flow through the whole body and thereby improving circulation to the sex organs. And there's evidence that they stimulate the release of endorphins, the body's "feel good" chemicals. So these peppers are often considered aphrodisiacs, especially for men.

However, the factor in chili peppers that causes the increased heart rate that brings on the improved circulation is called capsaicin, and it may be more irritating than pleasurable for some people. So those who have never tried chili peppers should test out their capacity for enjoying them before using them as a lovemaking enhancement.

Chili powder, which is pulverized from one or more varieties of hot chili peppers, is mentioned in the *Kama Sutra* as being one of five aphrodisiac spices.

Cinnamon

Used in Asia to ward off colds, cinnamon bark is appreciated worldwide for both its medicinal properties and as a flavoring for both savory and sweet dishes.

Although it produces heat in the body when ingested, cinnamon actually has anti-inflammatory properties and helps balance blood sugar. It's also often used in aromatherapy for relaxation and in massage oil for erotic stimulation.

Cloves

Cloves have a history as an aphrodisiac because the little nail-like dried buds and a part of the clove root are slightly phallic in form. Cloves, native to the Spice Islands of the Moluccas, were valued in Europe from about the 8th century on because of their sweet, spicy smell and taste. Like cinnamon and others of the sweeter smelling spices, they are used in cooking as well as in aromatherapy and erotic massage oil.

Clove oil contains the local anesthetic eugenol, used historically in dentistry, as well as salicylic acid, so it can be an effective painkiller. And when you're feeling no pain, you relax and become more ready for pleasure.

Coriander (Dried Cilantro Seed)

Coriander has a long history as a sexual stimulant and cure for impotence. Considered today to be a quick way for men to recover from a low sex drive, it was actually first prescribed as a sexual stimulant in ancient Egypt, where it was added to wine to increase a man's semen output. The ancient Chinese, who used it in love spells to cure impotence, also believed it could impart immortality to those who used it regularly. The ancient Greeks and Romans also added it to love potions, and the Greek physician Hippocrates is supposed to have created a drink that contained several pleasant spices including coriander that stimulated the libido so much it was banned.

Coriander is mentioned in the *Kama Sutra* as being one of five aphrodisiac spices. The medieval Arab classic *The Arabian Nights* also mentions it in a tale of a childless merchant whose 40 years of sexual inadequacy are cured by a concoction containing coriander. And the Bible compares the flavor of coriander to Manna.

Commonly used in curries, soups, stews, and pickles, coriander has a spicy citrus flavor.

Cumin

This spice is one of five mentioned in the *Kama Sutra* as having aphrodisiac powers, and in Arab countries, a paste made of ground cumin, pepper, and honey was used for purposes of sexual enhancement. In the Middle Ages, cumin seed also came to be a symbol of love and fidelity, an association that may have developed from the spice's earlier sexual associations.

High in iron, the little cumin seeds can give a body energy, enhanced immunity, good digestion, and possibly even protection against cancer. It's still prized in aphrodisiac cooking, especially in Middle Eastern countries, though it's also popular in Indian and Mexican cuisine.

Fennel

Fennel has a bold and powerful history, for in Greek mythology, Prometheus is supposed to have stolen fire from the gods with a stalk of the fennel plant. In addition, the wands of the followers of the Greek god Dionysus are believed to have come from the giant fennel plant, and as we know already, the Dionysian ceremonies were all about releasing sexual inhibitions. Fennel's use as an aphrodisiac dates to ancient Egypt where it was used for enhancing the libido. In the 1930s, this use was vindicated when researchers discovered fennel contained natural plant estrogens and has since proved to increase libido in both men and women.

Highly aromatic, fennel tastes similar to anise, and its bulb, seeds, and foliage have been used for culinary purposes around the world. However, fennel can be toxic in doses greater than a teaspoon—so be forewarned.

Mustard

The ancient Greeks were the first recorded culture to have used mustard as medicine, for they documented the ability of mustard to improve circulation. Its seeds have also been found in Egyptian tombs, suggesting they were another culture that may have had medical applications for this pungent plant. It's the heat of the ground seeds that gives the plant its reputation as an aphrodisiac for males, so by Medieval times it had become a forbidden food for monks, lest they be led astray after eating these pungent seeds. Indeed, the ancient Chinese thought mustard seeds' heat in the mouth was enough to effect the aphrodisiac response.

Good circulation, of course, offers the possibility of good sex, but mustard is also credited with causing increased adrenalin, which stimulates hormone production. In addition, mustard contains a fair amount of magnesium, manganese, selenium, zinc, and omega 3 fatty acids, all important nutrients for maintaining both good health and good sex. So have some mustard with your next hot dog.

Nutmeg and Mace

The nutmeg tree is an evergreen that's native to Indonesia's Spice Islands, though it has been used in India medicinally since 700 BCE and was prized by women in ancient China as an aphrodisiac. Both nutmeg and mace are derived from the same fruit, as nutmeg is the dried kernel, while mace is the dried shell from around the seed.

Nutmeg is sweeter and more aromatic than mace and has been used in love concoctions for centuries because it's believed to impart strength and enhanced libido, and research has shown that it does seem to increase the mating behaviors of laboratory mice.

But mace is also valued for its aphrodisiac properties, especially in Indian food, where it plays well with other spices in curry. In fact, curries are believed by their Indian cooks to be among the most aphrodisiac foods on the planet, thanks to the endorphins released in those consuming them.

Though it's a popular spice to include in pumpkin pies and is sold in your local grocery store, if taken in a large quantity, nutmeg can become hallucinogenic, and the same is true for mace. The culprits are the psychoactive properties of myristicin and elemicin, which are contained in both nutmeg and mace. In fact, recreational use of nutmeg has caused poisoning, and mace, though it has been used as a palliative for digestion as well as aches and pains, can cause vomiting, severe headaches, and tachycardia if taken in large doses. So while having them in quantities the size of small tins for your spice rack is safe, taking them in larger quantities is a bad idea.

Pimento/Allspice

The pimento tree, a tropical evergreen, is native to Central America, South America, the Caribbean Islands, Mexico, and the West Indies. Pimento is a stimulant that was commonly used in the folk medicine of ancient America. It's reputed to be an aphrodisiac when taken in large amounts.

The pimento received its name from early Spanish and Portuguese explorers, who thought its berries looked like peppercorns; "pimento" was their word for pepper. It's used both in cooking and for medicinal purposes.

Allspice, so called because its smell is like a combination of nutmeg, cinnamon, and cloves, comes from the spicy pimento berries, which when dried are ground to make allspice.

This spice has been a natural medical wonder; it relieves flatulence and is used to treat other digestive problems, such as stomach ache, indigestion, vomiting, diarrhea, colic, and dyspepsia. Its essential oil is used for all sorts of nervous disorders, from hysteria and convulsions to neuralgia, and when applied topically, it can relieve arthritis, muscle aches, chest infections, rheumatism, and bruises. Allspice has many antioxidants and is prescribed for colds and fever, diabetes, yeast and fungus infections, and menstrual cramps and bleeding. It's also been used by dentists as both an antiseptic and a local anesthetic.

Few natural remedies are constituted of so many helpful and palliative elements, for allspice has beta-carotene, vitamins A, B_1, B_2, B_3, and C, as well as minerals such as iron, selenium, manganese, potassium, and magnesium, and as we already know, all of these have positive effects on the sex organs, sex drive, circulation, and general health.

Though all of these positives may add to the belief in this spice as an aphrodisiac, the real reason is probably its luscious smell, which is like a delicious perfume that just makes you feel sexy.

Turmeric

This herb, also called *curcuma longa*, is in the ginger family and is often used in Indian curries and other types of Middle Eastern and Asian cuisine. Its rhizomes can be used fresh, but the more common way to use them is in their dried and powdered form, which has a deep orange-yellow color. Turmeric has a slightly peppery flavor and smells somewhat like mustard.

Turmeric is one of the five spices mentioned in the *Kama Sutra* as being highly aphrodisiac when ingested, and the essential oil version of turmeric is considered aphrodisiac when used in aroma therapy. So if you don't want to eat it, you can just sniff your way to a sexier life!

Saffron

Saffron, derived from the crocus flower, has a long-standing reputation as an aphrodisiac, and recent research has demonstrated that crocin, a carotenoid chemical found in crocus flowers, does indeed have aphrodisiac properties.

Saffron is the most expensive spice by weight—$1,000 per pound and up—and is graded by color, fragrance, and taste using very strict standards.

It is harvested from the stigma of the plant, and over 50,000 flowers are needed to produce that very expensive pound of saffron. But over the 3000 years of its cultivation, there has often been—and still is—a history of adulteration of various kinds, from mixing different grades together, to mixing in extraneous substances. Adulteration became so widespread in the Middle Ages in Europe that the Safranschou Code was implemented, under which a person could be fined, imprisoned, or executed for selling adulterated saffron.

Saffron has, of course, long been used in cooking and as a means of adding color to rice in Indian dishes, and it appears to assist with digestion and to improve mood. When its filaments are sun-dried, it's reputed to be a sexual stimulant for women. But note that while small doses can produce comfort and calm, large ones can be inebriating, Large doses are especially not recommended for those with mental problems or pregnant women because they can be toxic and possibly abortifacient.

Part VIII:
More Vegetative Matter

1. Flowers and Leaves

Albuca

In the villages around Chimoio in Central Mozambique, men usually have two to five wives. This plant is cultivated as an aphrodisiac, and the leaves are chewed by the men—presumably to help them keep up their end of the marriage bargain.

Damiana

A small shrub that grows best on rocky hills with lots of sun exposure, damiana is native to Mexico, Central America, southern California, and Texas. Its use as a sexual stimulant was first recorded by Spanish missionaries, who observed that the Indians of Mexico drank a tea brewed from damiana leaves for enhancing their sexual performance. It has been shown to be a good "pick-me-up" for sexually exhausted male rats, and female rats find it sexuality stimulating as well.

So a nice afternoon cuppa may be just what you need, but don't use it in Louisiana—it's a "prohibited plant" there.

Rose

Mentioned in the *Kama Sutra*, the scent of roses has been a part of the sexual seduction of women for centuries. However, Queen Cleopatra is supposed to have seduced Marc Antony with a concoction of rose, cinnamon, and cardamom, so apparently it works on men, too.

Red roses in particular, which came to the West from China, have been associated with love, fidelity, and passion, and came to be worn or carried at weddings to symbolize all these emotions. Sufi tradition elevates the scent as well as the flower to a symbol for divine love and transcendental desire. And there is some evidence that the scent of roses does have a real pharmacological effect in initiating pleasurable feelings similar to those of love.

Ginkgo Biloba

The ginkgo tree is both a "living fossil," with recognizable relatives dating back 270 million years, and an orphan, since it has no close living relatives. It predates flowering plants and produces seeds without flowers or fruit.

The nut-like inside of the seed is widely used in Asian cuisine, and extracts are derived from the leaves of the plant for medicinal purposes.

Gingko biloba's reputation is that it increases sexual energy. Its circulation enhancer supposedly increases blood flow to both the genitals and the brain, where in the latter, it enhances production of adrenaline, dopamine, and other neurotransmitters so the individual feels arousal, alertness, and pleasure.

Though over 40 components of the ginkgo tree have been identified, only two—flavonoids and terpenoids—seem to account for ginkgo's positive health benefits. Flavonoids are antioxidants, which have all the youth-retaining benefits of protecting the brain, nerves, blood vessels, heart, and retinas. Terpenoids dilate blood vessels and reduce platelet stickiness.

While Western doctors recommend ginkgo for maintaining circulation and memory, ordinary people are beginning to recognize that this plant's health benefits—especially those associated with the circulatory system—can be beneficial in treating erectile dysfunction.

Ylang-Ylang

The ylang-ylang, or cananga tree, is native to the Philippines and Indonesia, and commonly grown on South Pacific Islands. It is also grown in the Comoros Islands, where it accounts for 29% of the annual export of this poverty-stricken country.

The essential oils of ylang-ylang are used in aromatherapy. It blends well with other smells used in perfumes, and the oil derived from the flowers is used in many products such as Chanel No. 5.

As noted earlier, aromatherapy oils can enhance the desire for sex, and Margaret Mead in her studies of South Pacific Islanders made note of the use of ylang-ylang as an aphrodisiac.

2. Pulses

Pulses are grain legumes, which grow pods with seeds of various size, shape, and color. There are many categories of pulses, including dried beans, dried peas, chickpeas, lentils, and—if you do crossword puzzles—vetch.

Chickpeas, according to the *Kama Sutra*, can make a man ready to service a hundred women in a night—though we have to ask, should the chickpeas be turned into hummus first?

Also, green peas, according *The Perfumed Garden,* if they are boiled with onions and ground cinnamon, ginger, and cardamom, will bring passion and strength to coitus. However, all these other additives are also supposed to be aphrodisiacs, so the peas are surrounded by helpers in this particular dish.

Admittedly, most varieties of legumes, such as kidney, navy, red, and lima beans, are very rich in zinc, which as we already know, is important in the body's manufacture of hormones. And all legumes are high in fiber and protein, which are helpful in keeping us healthy. Black beans are high in folic acid, as well as the relaxation amino acid tryptophan. But the richest source of folic acid among legumes is in peanuts, which have loads of B vitamins as well as a lot of vitamin E, the sex hormone, helping both men and women with hormone manufacture.

Take *your* pulse after eating any of these pulses—if it's racing, you may be onto something!

Licorice

In China, licorice has been used as a medicine since ancient times. The plant is a legume, related to beans and peas, but its sweet flavor is extracted from the root. Licorice contains glycyrrhizin, which is fifty times sweeter than sugar, as well as essential oil, flavones, and tannins. Reputed to be good for the glands, especially the adrenals, whose health is essential for hormone production and libido, licorice is supposed to work particularly well for women, although one researcher showed that the smell of licorice was able to increase blood flow to male sex organs by 13 percent.

3. Coffee, Chocolate, and Vanilla

Coffee

Legend has it that humans in Ethiopia first began cultivating coffee trees when they noticed that their goats were mounting each other sexually after having eaten the coffee tree fruits and leaves. *Voila!* Coffee thereby had an instant reputation as an aphrodisiac.

However, as a morning brew to keep people awake during their working hours, we have to turn to the history of Arab scholars in Yemen, who were the first to record having boiled up a pot of coffee from roasted coffee beans. From there it made its way to Egypt and Turkey, and then around the world.

Caffeine is a well-known stimulant, and supposedly coffee has the same effect on women as oysters are said to have on men, i.e., it's a turn-on…and on, and on, and on.

Chocolate/Cocoa

The ancient Aztecs referred to chocolate as "the nourishment of the Gods," and the emperor Montezuma is said to have consumed large quantities of it (one source says 50 cups a day!) before engaging in sexual activity (he seems to have had a lot of concubines to service). In fact, it was a substance so prized by the Aztecs that their prostitutes were paid in cocoa. So perhaps Hersey has a *real* thing going with their chocolate kisses!

If you want to drink hot cocoa the way the ancient Central American Indians did, roast the cocoa beans and grind them up, then dissolve them in water with vanilla, ground cayenne pepper, diced pimento, ground cinnamon, and dried, ground squash seeds. If you like your cocoa sweet, then add honey to the mix.

Actually, cocoa contains small amounts of chemicals thought to affect neurotransmitters in the brain. One is tryptophan, a building block of serotonin, which really is a brain chemical involved in sexual arousal. Another is anandamide, which contributes to the euphoria of sexual pleasure. And yet another, phenethylamine, is related to amphetamine and is released in the brain when people feel desire. So when chocolate provides these chemicals, some attraction to another person may occur.

One other chemical in cocoa is theobromine, a mood-enhancing alkaloid similar to caffeine. So it makes us feel both good and perky. And dark chocolate has loads of antioxidants, so it takes out free radicals and helps us stay younger longer.

However, clinical studies so far have failed to show clearly a connection between chocolate consumption and arousal, so clinicians don't want to admit any real aphrodisiac powers for chocolate and prefer to say its effects may be psychological rather than physical. Nevertheless, chocolate contains more antioxidants than does red wine, and if you combine the two, you could be enhancing the youth-protecting powers of both. So have a little dark chocolate with a glass of Cabernet and just think, "I'm so sexy!"—it couldn't hurt!

Vanilla

Vanilla is native to Mesoamerica, although most of the world's supply of vanilla now comes from Madagascar and Tahiti. Vanilla takes months of curing and extensive hand-processing to develop the fragrance we know and love. Consequently, it is second only to saffron in cost, at $50-$200 per pound of beans.

The scent of vanilla has the reputation for increasing lust because it's one smell that seems to affect both genders. It has also been reported that if a man were to imbibe a shot of real vanilla extract an hour before having sex, he won't have to worry about impotence. If you're concerned about whether your vanilla extract is pure, you can make your own with Vodka and a couple of vanilla beans (though it will take a few days for the extract to be ready, so if you're in a hurry for the sex, try another route).

4. Rice, Wheat Germ, Soy, and Oats

Rice

All whole grains are supposed to be supportive of the libido, but rice is what has been traditionally thrown at weddings because it symbolizes fertility. In some Asian cultures, part of the marriage tradition involves the couple sharing a bowl of rice. And sake, which is wine made from rice, is supposed to have both the relaxation effects of alcohol combined with the excitement of rice's aphrodisiac properties.

Like many other whole grains, brown rice is very high in zinc, which has beneficial effects on the sex organs and hence boosts libido.

Wheat Germ

Wheat germ, its oil, and its sprouts have the reputation worldwide for strengthening the sex organs when eaten. One reason, at least for women, is that they contain estrogen and vitamin E—and both of these will help balance estrogen in the body. And we already know that vitamin E improves sex function and drive in both genders, so these components of wheat are good for everybody.

Soy

Soy in a variety of forms (kernels, milk, textured protein, powder, tofu, etc.) can boost sex health for women because it has a large amount of phytoestrogen. However, for women who have fought breast cancer that derived from excess estrogen in their systems, soy in the diet may be contraindicated, so it would be worthwhile checking with one's doctor before taking a daily dose. Also, be sure the soy product you're using hasn't been genetically modified. If the label doesn't tell you, keep looking for a product that does.

Oats

Eating refined oat cereal may not do much for your sex life, although it will probably fill up your tummy before you start your day. But another form of green or straw oats called Avena sativa does contain what seems to be a super sex enhancer. Scientists at San Francisco's nonprofit Institute for the Advanced Study of Human Sexuality did a six-week study of 40 research subjects and found that male testosterone levels increased 105 percent after they ingested Avena sativa, while men who had been impotent were able to perform again. Women in the study who had lost their sexual desire likewise experienced new levels of sexual interest after eating Avena sativa. And subjects also discovered other health benefits, including increased energy and endurance. So eating this oat grain may help increase a desire for sowing more wild oats!

Part IX:
Animal Proteins

1. Dairy and Meat

Cheese

Italian culture for centuries has believed cheese is an aphrodisiac, and many writers have associated its scent with sexuality. Cheese contains phenethylamine, which releases the same hormones as sexual pleasure—in fact, cheese contains ten times as much phenethylamine as does chocolate. Also, Dr. Max Lake, an Australian researcher, has shown that the five-carbon fatty acid that gives many cheeses their scent and flavor is closely related to a woman's mid-cycle vaginal pheromone. So when you want to eat something sexy, just say, "Cheese." And of course, you'll also be ready to have your picture taken!

Eggs

Eggs are among the world's most ancient fertility symbols, which is why bunnies (also symbols of fertility), deliver them in the spring. Whether we like it or not, Easter gets its name from the great goddesses of the ancient world, who traveled with the eggs and the bunnies to let their cultures know that spring, and the season of fertility and new life, had finally arrived. The yolk and white of an egg constitute a complete protein and are high in B_5, pantothenic acid, and B_6, pyridoxine, vitamins that assist in balancing hormone levels and fighting stress. And the cholesterol in eggs helps the female produce estrogen. Many people recommend eating raw chicken eggs before engaging in sex in order to increase stamina, and eggs are also believed by many to enhance one's libido. But all kinds of eggs, both fowl and fish, are considered to be aphrodisiac, which is why quail eggs and caviar are so prized.

Meat

Whether we're talking chicken, turkey, beef, or lamb, meat is full of protein, magnesium, zinc, and iron, all of which increase testosterone production. So, set up the barbeque, guys, and have a burger or chicken leg before that big game…or that hot date!

2. Seafood and Fish

As lovers of fish and seafood, we like to point out that the goddess of love, Aphrodite, was born of sea foam combined with the sperm from the great god Ouranos, whose son Chronos battled with his father, cut off his testicles, and threw them into the ocean. During the Renaissance, Botticelli painted *The Birth of Venus*, showing the beautiful goddess as she first sailed into port, nude and floating on a giant bivalve shell. This book's cover is a variation on that theme.

So here's a little tidbit about food and sex for you: in the ancient world, fish was considered a sacred food, eaten only on the day dedicated to the goddess, which in almost every culture at that time was Friday (the female goddess equivalent to Aphrodite/Venus got only one day of the seven-day week—the male gods got all the rest). Anyway, on the day dedicated to the goddess, Friday, people were allowed to eat fish in a ritual meal. And when the Jews were forced to live in Babylonia during their Babylonian Captivity, they were introduced to the eating of fish on Friday. They subsequently brought this tradition of a Friday fish meal back with them, and it eventually got passed on to the Catholic Church when that organization came to power. But almost nobody today knows that when they go out for fish on Friday, they're celebrating a tradition begun as a ritual for the great goddesses of love and sex of the ancient world.

Below we discuss the benefits of eating oysters and mussels, but all fish and seafood contribute to this tradition of love because they're rich in protein, B vitamins, and omega-3 fatty acids, which heal the nerves, boost blood circulation, and are excellent at maintaining reproductive health.

If you don't like fish or seafood, just remember: Aphrodite is watching!

Eel

The Japanese love freshwater eel, known as unagi eel, and it's often found in American sushi restaurants, grilled and served with a sweet sauce and sesame seeds. What most sushi establishments won't say is that this kind of eel is considered to be an aphrodisiac.

Eel is high in vitamins A, B_1, B_2, B_{12}, D, and E, and it's used in Japan and some parts of Europe as a natural anti-aging nutritional supplement. Unfortunately, unagi eel has been over-fished and recently put on the endangered list, so maybe you should consider other aphrodisiac foods instead, at least for a while.

Mussels

Like the oyster, mussels have a long history of being eaten for their aphrodisiac qualities. And this is with good reason, since studies show these little critters release estrogen *and* testosterone. So maybe you really can build your sexual muscles by enjoying some mussels steamed in a buttery white wine sauce.

Oysters

Juvenal, the second century Roman comic playwright, seems to have been the first to make a written claim for oysters as an aphrodisiac food, for in his satire he joked how women would become wanton after drinking wine and eating oysters. But while oysters are supposed to resemble the female genitalia, they do have a high content of zinc and protein, both of which contribute to production of testosterone and healthy sperm, as well as taurine, an amino acid that affects the heart. So men sometimes take oyster extract to improve their sexual endurance. Perhaps they've learned Casanova claimed he ate 50 raw oysters a day to improve *his* endurance.

Maybe Juvenal had the basics right about oysters being an aphrodisiac food—he was just making jokes about the wrong gender!

Part X:
Alcohol

Absinthe

"Absinthe makes the heart grow fonder," was a phrase Honora heard first while she was visiting New Orleans at the age of 16. She got the pun, but she didn't really understand that the point of it was to credit absinthe as an aphrodisiac.

The question remains today as to what exactly in the pretty green drink, known to those who adore it as "the green fairy," makes it so addictive and gives those who drink it the mind-altering effects they report?

Science has yet to determine the exact reason it shifts reality so effectively—and yes, makes those who indulge experience altered sensations of a synesthetic kind that can include sexual highs. One factor has to be that the wormwood from which absinthe is made contains thujone, which is similar to marijuana's THC, but that may not be the whole answer. There's no question, though, that as long as those who imbibe it stay awake and aware and want to enhance their drinking experience with sex and their sexual experience with the drink, they're likely to succeed.

Agave

Agave nectar, which is a sweet juice from the core of varieties of the agave plant, has the reputation of also being an aphrodisiac. This may be because the darker versions of this sweetener are rich in vitamins and minerals and are a good substitute for syrup on pancakes and waffles, or more likely, it's because some varieties of the agave plant are fermented to create alcoholic drinks, such as agave wine, tequila, and mezcal. When these drinks were first introduced, they were referred to as *aguardiente*, which literally translates as "water with teeth."

It isn't known whether the people of Mexico had fermented alcoholic drinks before the Spanish Conquest, but there's a myth associated with agave drinks that says a lightning bolt struck an agave plant, cooking it and breaking it open, thus making the liquid inside available for humans to enjoy. Because of this mythical beginning from on high, the agave drinks are called "the elixir of the gods" in Mexico.

Wine

Grapes are rich in antioxidants, and so is the wine that comes from the grapes. Acknowledged in both the Old and the New Testaments, wine has an unbeatable religious heritage as a beverage. A glass or two of wine can greatly enhance romance because wine relaxes us and helps to increase other sense experiences.

Drinking red wine, if one isn't allergic to it, can be a sensual experience in itself, because the color is luscious (red being often associated with sexuality) and the taste is delicious. And wine glasses are meant to be fondled and caressed, even before one begins to do the same to one's partner. Also, red wine has resveratrol, which has been shown to have cancer-fighting properties, lowers levels of bad cholesterol, lowers levels of blood sugar, appears to be anti-inflammatory, and may have heart-health benefits.

Always remember, though, that a little wine may contribute to sexual arousal, but too much can put an end to what might have been a pleasurable encounter.

Part XI:
A Few Other Foods of Interest

Honey

The ancient Egyptians based many of their medicines on honey, and this included cures for impotence and sterility. And according to legend, the Greek god Eros (Cupid) dipped the tips of his arrows in honey before shooting them into the hearts of potential lovers.

Because raw honey provides a healthy, natural boost to energy, it's recommended today as an adjunct to many other healing remedies. In terms of its efficacy in improving sex, it does contain boron, which assists in regulating testosterone and estrogen, as well as B vitamins, phytochemicals, and enzymes. Of course, honey is the product of bees who are harvesting flower nectar and taking it back to their hive to feed newborn baby bees, so really, honey is all about sex. After all, isn't our first introduction to sex supposed to be a discussion of "the birds and the bees"?

The earliest fermentation of wine, based on prehistoric evidence going back to approximately 9000 BCE, used honey as a part of the process, and mead, also called "honey wine," has been with us ever since. Its first historic description was in a hymn of the Rig-Veda, one of the sacred books of ancient India, dating somewhere between 1700 and 1100 BCE, and Aristotle wrote about it in the 4th century BCE when it was the preferred drink during the Golden Age of Greece. It seems to have been particularly popular in the Middle Ages, when Beowulf and his cronies drank it in their mead halls, and newlyweds drank it on their "honeymoon" to sweeten their new marriage.

Kelp

The lowly seaweed known as kelp turns out to be rich in lots of vitamins, minerals, and other nutrients, and particularly iodine, necessary for health of the thyroid gland, the proper functioning of which contributes to sex drive and physical energy. Perhaps this is why in some parts of the planet, and especially in Asian countries, kelp is valued as an aphrodisiac. So next time you need some sexual help, try kelp.

Mushrooms

In ancient Egypt, mushrooms were believed to impart immortality, while in other cultures, certain species of mushrooms, like peyote, were valued for the hallucinogenic effects they'd bring on.

A legend from the South Pacific tells of women who wandered in the island forests, searching for food, and when they sampled certain types of fungi, they began experiencing sexual ecstasy. Today, shitake mushrooms, which are touted for reducing cholesterol, protecting against cancer, and preventing infection and inflammation, have this same reputation as an aphrodisiac, particularly in Asian countries, where women eat them to become more sexually responsive. We never knew before that a fungus could be so much fun!

Sauerkraut

This fermented cabbage product has oodles of vitamins, minerals, calcium, and fiber, is good for the digestion, contains a property that fights cancer—and on top of other benefits, sauerkraut boosts libido. Try some next time you eat a long German sausage, and you'll wonder which one is the best aphrodisiac.

Spirulina

Spirulina, also known as blue-green algae, has the reputation for enhancing male libido because it improves circulation, so it's commonly used as an over-the-counter adjunct to erectile dysfunction. Sometimes referred to as a "superfood," it's rich in protein, vitamins, minerals and beta-carotene. It was used by the Aztecs and Incas because it offers tremendous nutrition in small amounts. Of course, anything this nutritious is bound to be good for women, too.

Truffles

The truffle is an underground fungus that grows close to the roots of trees. Since the truffle isn't a spice, its price isn't compared to spice items such as saffron, But black truffles, sometimes nicknamed black diamonds, sell for $1,200 a pound, and white truffles can bring in $7,000 per pound.

A 3.3 pound white truffle sold at a charity auction for $330,000 in 2007. The fellow who dished out that amount for this tasty fungus, a casino billionaire, matched his own record in 2010, paying the same amount for a pair of white truffles, one of which weighed nearly two pounds.

Prized for its rarity, the truffle was considered an aphrodisiac in ancient Greece and Rome. Its musky scent, which is said to replicate that of male pheromones, is supposed to increase the sensitization of the skin—and presumably lure women in for a petting session! In the Arab world after it embraced Islam, truffles were not permitted to be sold near mosques because it was feared the Muslim populace might be morally corrupted by eating them.

Napoleon, on the other hand, didn't mind their corrupting influence and ate them to enhance his male potency.

Aphrodisiacs: Incredible Edibles for Better Sex

Both black and white truffles have the aphrodisiac reputation, so if you can afford them without selling your farm or first-born child, go ahead and indulge.

Part XII:
Some Not So Common Plants with an Aphrodisiac History

Acorus Calamus (also known as Sweet Flag)

Calamus is generally thought to be indigenous to most of Asia, although it has been introduced to Europe, South Africa, Australia, and North America. Its leaves and rhizomes have been used traditionally for perfumes, and its dried rhizomes have also been used as substitutes for sweet spices such as ginger, nutmeg, and cinnamon.

Among several Native American tribes, the calamus plant was considered a ward against illness of various kinds, as well as a healer and protector.

In ancient Asia and Egypt, this rhizome was believed to be a powerful aphrodisiac. In Europe it was sometimes added to wine, and its root may have been an ingredient in absinth. Traditionally, it has been thought that when calamus root is added to a bath, it can create sexual stimulation.

Asafoetida

Reputedly used in Ayurvedic medicine as a sexual stimulant, asafoetida is the dried gum oleoresin from the underground rhizome of several species of Ferula, a herb native to Afghanistan but cultivated in India. It has an odor similar to leeks when it is cooked.

Ashwagandha/Withania Somnifera

Withania somnifera is also known as ashwagandha, Indian ginseng, poison gooseberry, and winter cherry. A member of the nightshade family, it is reputed to be India's most potent hot plant, and according to one source, it is used in Ayurvedic medicine to improve low libido and sexual function by both men and women. Its primary chemical components are alkaloids and steroidal lactones.

Ashwagandha is a Sanskrit word meaning "horse's smell" because the plant's root presumably smells like a sweaty horse. The word *somnifera* is Latin for "sleep inducing."

Catuaba

The name *catuaba* is applied to infusions of the bark of several trees native to Brazil. The name in Guarani means "what gives strength to the Indian." An infusion of the bark has been used in the traditional medicine of the Tupi Indians of Brazil as both an aphrodisiac and a stimulant of the central nervous system, and it has been suggested that a group of three alkaloids are responsible for these reported results.

Catuaba bark and its preparations are sold in health food stores as sexual stimulants and remedies for erectile dysfunction. Native healers also prescribe it to counter anxiety, memory loss, and insomnia.

Cistanche

This herb has been used in Chinese medicine for centuries as a blood tonic, brain tonic, and sex tonic. Claims are made that it can remedy impotence and premature ejaculation and increase fertility of both genders.

Cnidium Seeds

Cnidium, a plant found in China and Oregon, has been a staple of traditional Chinese medicine for millennia. Though its principal use has been for skin conditions, the seeds are also used for treatment of erectile dysfunction, infertility, sexual performance, and sex drive.

Durian Fruit

Again, this is a food you probably won't find in your local grocery store, but it's a big seller in Malaysian countries, where it's reputed to have aphrodisiac qualities. Regarded by some as the "king of fruits," the durian is quite large, has a strong odor, and is covered with sharp, spiky thorns.

The odor of the durian is distinctive, and though some find it fragrant, others think it's disgusting. Because the latter seem to be in the majority, the fruit has been banished from certain classier hotels and public transportation in Southeast Asia. However, among the Javanese, it's still widely prized for its touted aphrodisiac qualities. And the Malaysians have a saying: "When the durians fall, the sarongs rise."

Guarana

Growing in the Amazon rainforest, the red fruit of the guarana plant has a long history in the folklore of the Amazonian natives because of the black eyes that appear as the fruit ripens. Both the fruit and its seeds are used in native folk medicine for weight balancing, pain killing, calming nerves, increasing energy, and stimulating libido. In Brazil, guarana is used also as a remedy for headaches, fatigue, and slowing the aging process.

Horny Goat Weed

The genus of this flowering plant is Epimedium, of which there are about 60 species in the family Berberidaceae, most of which are endemic to southern China. It is also known by such colorful names as barrenwort, bishop's hat, fairy wings, rowdy lamb herb, randy beef grass, and yin yang huo.

The aphrodisiac benefits attributed to it are primarily for men, including a reversing of erectile dysfunction, improved testosterone production, increased sperm production, a stimulation of sex drive and activity, and increased energy.

The legend associated with the aphrodisiac effect of this herb is that it was discovered by a Chinese goatherd who noticed increased sexual activity in the flock after they ate the leaves of the plant. It has been shown that these effects are the result of the plant's content of icariin, a flavonol, which is used in Western medicine to improve sexual response and treat impotence.

Huanarpo Macho

Believed by the people of Brazil to be able to stimulate male sexual response, and known in Peru as Peruvian Viagra, huanarpo macho is a plant covered with beautiful red-orange blooms that grows in the Amazon Maranon River Valley. Since one of its scientific names is *Jatropha aphrodisiaca*, one would certainly think its aphrodisiac reputation surely has something behind it. Indeed, it has been used in South American folk medicine for both premature ejaculation and erectile dysfunction, though it has other medicinal uses as well, including calming nerves and increasing energy.

Muira Puama

Muira puama is a small tree native to the Brazilian Amazon. Also called "potency wood," its bark and root have been used by indigenous peoples in the treatment of sexual debility, as well as fatigue, rheumatism, and neuromuscular problems. The Institute of Sexology in Paris, France, has done clinical studies on the efficacy of muira puama in treating libido loss with some reported positive results. Herbalists in the United States are currently using muira puama extracts to treat patients for sexual improvement, PMS, and menstrual cramps, as well as nervous system disorders. The extracts also appear to have mood-enhancing capabilities. But because of the plant's many constituents, it is hard to pinpoint the chemicals that are responsible for the results.

Reported side effects appear to include insomnia when the extract is taken in high doses.

Picho Huayo

Picho huayo is a tree that grows both in the rainforests of the Amazon and the cloud forests of the Andes. The leaves and fruit of the tree are used medicinally to treat many ailments, including colds, fevers, high blood pressure, and snake-bite, and in addition they are popular in love potions, which men rub themselves with in the belief it will make them irresistible to women.

Rhodiola Rosea

Rhodiola rosea, a herb that grows in the arctic, has been studied at Columbia University, where research has shown it appears to enhance libido, performance, orgasm, and energy in both genders, as well as improving stamina in men and counteracting the effects of menopause in women. It may also improve mood, counter depression, reduce fatigue, and improve both mental and physical performance. However, at the current time, there is scientific acceptance only for treatment of depression in humans.

Russia and Scandinavia have used Rhodiola rosea for centuries to deal with the cold climate and stress of life. It has also been used in traditional Chinese medicine. Nevertheless, studies have shown that the chemical composition of the plant varies in different parts of the world.

Rosewood Oil

Oil produced by the rosewood tree, which is native to the Amazon rainforest, is highly appreciated in South America as an aphrodisiac for countering frigidity in women, as well as for healing acne, curing headaches, and reducing fevers. Unfortunately, a recent upsurge in the commercial use of rosewood oil means an increased felling of the trees, which may bring damage to the rainforest bioregion, so it is probably wise to consider alternatives to this treatment.

Tamamuri

A member of the mulberry family, the tamamuri tree grows in the Peruvian Amazon where the native inhabitants believe that eating the white sap that comes from the tree's punctured bark will increase a male's ability to father male children. The tree bark is also used medicinally by the native people to eliminate bacteria, yeast, and fungi; soothe pain; and even kill cancer.

Associated with magical properties, the bark is also used by native medical practitioners as a treatment for syphilis. As an aphrodisiac, the bark is turned into a tonic and drunk to stimulate sexual function.

Tongkat Ali

Eurycoma longifolia (commonly called tongkat ali) is a flowering plant in the family Simaroubaceae, native to Indonesia, Malay, Java, Thailand, Vietnam, and Laos. Many of the common names refer to the plant's medicinal use and extreme bitterness. Though there are reputed traditional medical uses for the plant, such as its effectiveness in treating malaria, tumors, ulcers, diabetes, and cancer, it is generally believed that most Southeast Asians use it for sexual purposes, such as the increase of male virility and prowess.

A large number of products sold as Eurycoma longifolia over the internet and in some markets have turned out to be fakes, and some products are reputedly contaminated, so let the buyer beware.

Tribulus Terrestris

Tribulus terrestris is a taprooted herbaceous perennial found growing in colder climates as a summer annual. About a week after its flowers bloom, they become fruits that in short order fall apart into four or five spiky nutlets that have two or three very sharp spines. Its name originated in Greek and means "water chestnut," which was translated into Latin as "tribulos." The Latin word "tribulus" meant a caltrop or spiky weapon, but even in classical times, the word also came to mean this plant as well.

An extract of the plant has been claimed to increase the body's natural testosterone levels and build strength and muscle, though it has failed to do so in controlled studies with humans. However, the plant has long been used in Indian Ayurvedic tonics, as well as in Unani, another Indian medical system.

In animal studies, Tribulus terrestris has proved to enhance sexual behavior, apparently by stimulating the brain's androgen receptors. It is currently being touted as a promoter of increased sex drive, though the research for this claim was again with animal subjects.

Other animal studies have demonstrated that administering the extract of Tribulus terrestris could produce statistically significant levels of male sexual hormones suggestive of aphrodisiac activity, although other studies with humans have failed to provide similar results.

Part XIII:
Psychotropic Aphrodisiacs

The strongest aphrodisiacs are poisonous, some of them hallucinogenic or psychotropic, and overdoses can cause death. If you choose to sample them, do so with caution. Remember that herbs are unprocessed drugs and can potentially interact with other medications.

It is strictly for your edification that we include the following list of alleged aphrodisiacs—whether they might actually have the power to produce aphrodisiac experiences is not known; what is known is that they can be toxic and must be treated with gravity.

And while all the recipes in our "Killer Cookbooks"[3] are non-toxic and delectable, an aspiring mystery writer might consider one of these psychotropic aphrodisiacs as part of a potential plot.

Belladonna

Known as the "witch's plant," belladonna is a nightshade and a sister of the mandrake. The entire plant contains very strong alkaloids and hence is hallucinogenic. Though it purports to increase sexual desire, an overdose can lead to death from paralysis of the respiratory system.

Betel Palm Seeds

A traditional aphrodisiac in Ayurvedic medicine, betel palm seeds contain alkaloids that can have a strong stimulating effect on the whole body.

----

[3] The three Ariel Quigley Mysteries and Cookbooks (each combined into one easy to handle paperback) are available at Amazon and on Kindle. (www.arielquigleymysteries.com)

Borrachero

Native to Colombia, this plant's leaves can be made into a decoction that is highly intoxicating and disorienting. Though it is used as an aphrodisiac, borrachero contains tropane alkaloids, with a high percentage of scopolamine, which even in small doses can lead to hallucinations, paranoid behavior, and delusions.

Datura

Datura stramonium, which is also known by the common names of Jimson weed, loco weed, and sometimes Thorn Apple and Angel's Trumpet, is a plant in the nightshade family that probably originated in the Americas but is now grown worldwide.

Used in herbal medicine as an analgesic and also to relieve asthma, the plant contains tropane alkaloids and is often considered a magical agent, used in spiritual, entheogenic rituals for the purpose of achieving visions. These alkaloids are highly hallucinogenic and delirium producing and can be toxic and even fatal in doses higher than those prescribed for medical usage.

Hawaiian Baby Woodrose

This plant is a climbing vine that was originally indigenous to the subcontinent of India, but it has been introduced to many other environments worldwide, including Hawaii, the Caribbean, and Africa. It has been used as a stimulant for women, as well as in magical love potions. Its seeds contain the ergoline alkaloids ergine and lysergic acid amide which can engender a euphoric psychedelic effect, while an aphrodisiac effect has also been reported. This is a plant whose hallucinogenic effects were not recognized until the 1960s.

Kava

Kava (*Piper methysticum*, meaning "intoxicating pepper") comes from Polynesia, and its reputation as an aphrodisiac appears to derive from its ability to relax anxiety and reduce stress while allowing the individual's mind to remain clear. Pharmacological studies have shown that kava contains at least 15 kavalactones, all of which are psychoactive. Kava has been used traditionally for a variety of medicinal treatments, many of them related to sexual dysfunction.

If the rhizome of the kava plant is macerated, combined with coconut milk, and fermented, it is reputed to become psychotropic and to increase in its aphrodisiac qualities.

Mandrake Root

Mandrake root as a magical plant is widely known today thanks to the Harry Potter book and film in which mandrake plants were found in the greenhouse at Hogwarts. However, its use as an aphrodisiac goes back millennia to ancient Mesopotamia, Egypt, Cyprus, and Greece, where it was associated with the powers of the goddesses of love in those cultures. It was also described as a sexual stimulant by the Greek doctor Theophrastus in the third century BCE.

According to the Old Testament Book of Genesis (30: 14-16), Jacob's son Reuben found some mandrakes in a field of wheat and brought them to his mother, Leah, whose barren sister Rachel prevailed upon her to give them to her, believing the mandrake would help her become pregnant. The Greek Orthodox Church forbade its members to use mandrake root for fear it would lead them into rampant promiscuity.

The power of the mandrake to enchant the minds of humans is evidenced by how often it has been referenced in literature: by

Shakespeare in *Othello, Antony and Cleopatra, Romeo and Juliet,* and *Henry IV, Part II*, as well as by John Donne, Samuel Beckett, John Steinbeck, and Terry Pratchett—and of course, J.K. Rowling in the Harry Potter book mentioned above.

Native to the entire Mediterranean area, mandrake was thought to cause madness if not used properly. Because the root is shaped like a little human, it was also believed to contain a spirit that would shriek when the root was pulled out of the ground; if the harvester heard the scream, he or she would die from the experience. Hence, a dog was often tied to the plant and enticed with meat that was placed just out of reach to pull up the root while the human harvester ran far enough away he or she wouldn't hear the scream.

Oddly, in spite of the negatives associated with its reputation, the mandrake was also believed to bring prosperity, health, fertility, and protection if placed on the mantel, tied to the head of one's bed, or carried on the person.

Like belladonna, mandrake was believed to be a "witches' plant" during the Middle Ages when it was supposedly used in flying ointments. Containing several hallucinogenic tropane alkaloid substances, such as atropine, apoatropine, hyoscyamine, and scopolamine, mandrake is one of the nightshades, is highly psychotropic, and can cause delirium, coma, and even death if used improperly in high doses.

Morning Glory Seeds

First used in China as medicine for their laxative properties, morning glory seeds contain ergoline alkaloids that are strongly psychedelic when taken in large doses, similar to the results of LSD. This is why the morning glory was called the "plant of prophecy" and used in pre-Columbian times for religious and divinatory purposes. The seeds were also ingested to help women overcome gynecological problems, but because they contain lysergic acid, they can also cause uterine contractions.

In addition to the care that must be taken not to overindulge in the seeds themselves because of their alkaloid content, it is hard to find seeds that have not been treated with methylmercury or pesticides, which can cause neural damage or liver problems if ingested.

Passion Flowers and Passion Fruits

Passiflora, known also as passion flowers or passion vines, is a genus of about 500 species of plants, the leaves and roots of which were long used by Native American people of South America and later by European colonists. Leaves and fruits were used medicinally to make a tea for killing pain as well as for treatment of various ailments, including hysteria, epilepsy, and insomnia. The dried leaves are also often smoked.

The fruit, eaten as is or used as a sweetener in many countries and cultures around the world, sounds as if it should have a sexual association, but the name of the plant was designated by Spanish missionaries, who thought the flowers resembled Christ's crown of thorns, which was placed on his head during his passion and crucifixion.

Many species of this plant contain alkaloids, and though the flower and fruit have only traces, the leaves and roots have been used for mind-altering purposes. Other compounds found in some varieties of the plants make them somewhat poisonous.

The *Passiflora incarnata* has demonstrated sex-enhancing results in laboratory mice, which registered higher sperm counts. However, its potential side effects include toxicity, dizziness, lack of coordination, mental confusion, blood vessel inflammation, and altered consciousness. It is definitely not safe to ingest during pregnancy as it can cause uterine contractions.

Poppy Seeds

Thanks to the fact that the 1939 film *The Wizard of Oz* has been watched by more people on the planet than any other, most of us know by now that a species of the poppy flower is the source of opium and can put people to sleep.

However, poppy seeds are also good nutrition, providing flavor to muffins, bagels, and even salad dressings. Full of B vitamins and linoleic acid, they are used in the medicine of Iran and Algeria as an analgesic and in Indian Ayurveda as an aphrodisiac.

Because the seeds of the poppy contain both codeine and morphine, ancient Egyptian doctors gave them to their patients to relieve pain. For this same reason, consuming large amounts of poppy seeds can cause hallucinations.

Prickly or Mexican Poppy

This plant has a narcotic effect and is sometimes smoked as an alternative to cannabis. Among the Mayan and Aztec people, it was considered as an analgesic and an aphrodisiac, as well as being used by the Aztecs in ritual sacrifice ceremonies. It is also reputed that Chinese residents in Mexico manufactured a product from the plant that was similar to opium.

The seeds of the plant contain 22-36 percent of a non-edible oil with toxic alkaloids. In India it's known for its psychoactive properties; it's listed as poisonous in *Poisonous Plants of the United States* because it's fatal to birds, and cattle who eat the plant can pass toxic alkaloids to the unsuspecting in their milk.

Sassafras

Indigenous to North America, sassafras leaves were used as a spice by the Native Americans, for whom tradition says the sassafras tree was a "love tree." This culinary use was adopted by the Creole cooks of Louisiana for their gumbo recipes. Also, for many years, sassafras was used as the principle flavoring in root beer and was also used as a tea, until the FDA banned its use because of its potential for contributing to cancer.

The essential oil of the sassafras tree is safrole, once used extensively in soaps and perfumes. However, safrole has more recently been used in the street manufacture of MDMA, known as "ecstasy," and of the drug MDA.

Ingestion of the oil or its use in erotic massage may bring about psychedelic experiences or unwanted toxic side effects.

Spanish Fly

Probably one of the most famous—and destructive—supposed aphrodisiacs is Spanish fly. It is made from a species of blister beetle that coats its eggs with a substance called cantharidin, which induces blisters and is comparable as a poison to strychnine. The entire beetle, which contains about five percent cantharidin in its body, is dried and crushed to produce the Spanish fly powder. When the powder is ingested, the body excretes the cantharidin in the urine, causing irritation and burning in the urogenital tract and swelling of the genitals. This physical reaction was once thought to be sexual arousal and led to the idea that Spanish fly had aphrodisiac qualities.

However, cantharidin is highly toxic, inflaming the kidneys and possibly damaging them permanently, as well as causing gastrointestinal disturbances, convulsions, and even death. Ergo, Spanish fly is not an aphrodisiac—it is a poison that can be deadly.

Wild Lettuce

Wild lettuce has the scientific name *Lactuca virosa*, which was used in Europe and North America as a narcotic and sexual stimulant. It includes about a hundred wild and domestic species, though very few are native to North America. Through a process of blending in a blender and then drying of the plant's liquefied leaves, a dried residue can be placed in an opium pipe and smoked like marijuana. The resulting experience is described as intoxication of a mild form, although smoking large quantities can be toxic.

Wild lettuce was used in medicine and ritual in ancient Egypt, where it was associated with Min, the god of fertility, whose effigy was placed in a patch of wild lettuce during his festivals. Wild lettuce was also used as an aphrodisiac in Egypt, though the Egyptians were warned that too much of a good and pleasurable thing might dull the brain.

By contrast, the Greeks used wild lettuce as an anaphrodisiac, giving it to their priests to cool their sexual desires.

Wild lettuce is often ingested for its mild psychotropic effects, which are described as similar to the smoking of opium. It arrived in the United States after the American Revolution, and in 1792 a Philadelphia doctor wrote about its opium-like qualities. In recent times, it has been valued as a marijuana substitute.

Though wild lettuce is seldom used today in herbal medicine, it is known to be useful as a sedative for insomnia, anxiety, tension, and nervousness. It is sometimes used as an aid to meditation. It is also sometimes recommended to treat premature ejaculation. Though its effects are not described as being as virulent as most of the substances in this section, it is important for the reader to be aware of its psychotropic potential.

Yohimbine

In Africa, yohimbe bark extract has traditionally been used both as an herbal aphrodisiac and in a prescription drug used for erectile dysfunction in men. It comes from the stripped bark of a West African evergreen tree.

Yohimbine is an alkaloid of yohimbe and its main active ingredient; it is also found naturally in *Rauwolfia serpentina* (Indian Snakeroot), along with several other alkaloids. Yohimbine has both stimulant and aphrodisiac effects and is sold as a prescription medicine for treating sexual dysfunction; the NIH states it has been shown effective in human studies for treating male impotence and orgasmic dysfunction, as well as for treating reduced libido in women.

However, it can both increase blood pressure when used in small amounts and cause low blood pressure when used in large amounts, and unfortunately, the range between an effective dose and a dangerous dose is quite narrow. Too high a dosage can lead to rapid heart rate, headaches, dizziness, panic attacks, insomnia, hallucinations, heart attacks, paralysis, or even death. It should not be taken by anyone suffering from liver, kidney, or heart problems or any psychological disorders.

Part XIV:
In Conclusion

Michel Foucault in *The History of Sexuality* says that Western culture has for centuries been fixated on sexuality. The social convention of treating sex as something to be hidden because it is unclean has created a discourse *around* it, which would not have been the case if it had been considered natural.

In cultures where it has for centuries been considered natural instead of shameful, like China, Japan, and India, it has been treated as "*Ars Erotica*," sex practiced as an erotic art.

In Western culture, however, because it is believed to be something dirty, sex has for generations been seen as "*Scientia Sexualis*," the science of sex, where people have become fixated on finding out the "truth" about sex and then confessing it at every opportunity. And when one believes that any act one desires to do would be condemned if others knew about it, then one *must* find a confessor, either a trusted friend, a spiritual mentor, or a paid psychiatric listener, to whom one then confesses the "truth."

Of course, if one is committing an act that others might condemn (because having sex is often referred to as "doing the nasty"), then there is never any way for one to "get it right."

And so, dear reader, if you are among the many whom Western culture has influenced in this way, we urge you to relax. Take a tip from Eastern cultures: focus on giving your partner a good time, and turn the experience into an erotic art. And a really easy way to do this is to start in the kitchen, create something delicious, feed it enticingly to your beloved, and then work your way to the bedroom. Enjoy the feast!

About the Authors

Honora Finkelstein has been an intelligence officer with the U.S. Navy, a small-press publisher, a technical writer, and a prize-winning features editor for Arundel Communications in Northern Virginia. She has been widely published in newspapers, magazines, and journals, has co-authored two nonfiction books, and has taught futurist and self-development workshops across the United States, in Canada, and in Europe. She was a workshop director for the International Women's Writing Guild for 15 years, a contributing editor to Pathways Magazine in Washington, D.C. for 25 years, has a Ph.D. in English, and has taught Western culture, literature, and writing at several universities.

Her interest in metaphysical subjects goes back to childhood when she had her first out-of-body experience while learning to tie her shoes. In the 1990s she produced and hosted a talk show on self-development and futurist topics called *Kaleidoscope for Tomorrow* on community cable television in Fairfax, Virginia, an experience that qualified her as an "agent provocateur."

She is the author of *Magicians*, a futurist look at what might happen in our culture if a small group of dedicated people devoted themselves to making positive change happen. To the embarrassment of some of her more traditional friends and academic colleagues, she also does past-life and Tarot card readings and occasionally talks to ghosts.

Susan Smily, during her 25 years in the classroom, was an author, publisher, and workshop leader in elementary science education in Canada, Australia, and the United States (acquiring a gray hair for every student she taught). She created her own business for the development and production of a wide range of elementary education materials, worked as a writer, editor, and consultant with several educational programs, and made presentations at over 40 school and district professional development days. She was also once the Science Teacher of the Year (cover girl) for Boreal Science Supply Catalog and as a result had coffee stains on her face in every high school in Canada.

She is the author of "Pianissimo," a one-act play that was presented off Broadway on April 13-15, 1998, at the Festival of Collective Voices, Harold Clurman Theatre in New York.

She has traveled extensively in North America, Europe, Australia, and the Far East. She developed an interest in metaphysical studies in the early 1990s and has since become involved in studying many areas of spirituality, including Native American, Vedanta, and Kabbalah. She is also an energy reader and "psychic diagnostician."

Finkelstein and Smily have appeared on panels at numerous mystery writers' conferences and have spoken to groups at libraries, arts centers, and Kiwanis Clubs across the U.S. and Canada. They are the winners of the 2007 Love Is Murder Readers' Choice Award (the Lovey) for Best First Novel for *The Chef Who Died Sautéing,* as well as awards from the Public Safety Writers Association for their thriller *Walk-In* and for *The Reporter Who Died Probing.*

Honora Finkelstein and Susan Smily

Our Books

The Ariel Quigley Mystery Series
by Honora Finkelstein and Susan Smily

The Chef Who Died Sautéing & A Killer Cookbook #1

The Lawyer Who Died Trying & A Killer Cookbook #2

The Reporter Who Died Probing & A Killer Cookbook #3
Available on Amazon as paperbacks and eBooks
Second Editions, El Amarna Publishing, April, 2012
The novels were previously published by Hilliard and Harris Publishing, and the cookbooks were previously published by Fenton Press.
* * *

Walk-In
A thriller by Honora Finkelstein and Susan Smily
Oak Tree Press, February, 2012
* * *

Magicians: A Novel of Transformation and Co-Creation
Honora Finkelstein
El Amarna Publishing, October, 2011
* * *

A collection of poetry *by Honora Finkelstein*
I Am Anima: Songs of Yin Energy
Kundalini Rising: Songs of Power and Spirit
Syzygy: Songs for Fools and Magicians
* * *

Cross-Currents
A neo-noir novel by Powell Smily
realized by Susan Smily and Honora Finkelstein
El Amarna Publishing, April, 2012
* * *

ScienceWorks: A Guide to Science Instruction...with a Difference!
by Susan Smily, with drawings by Louaynne Rhode
* * *

All books are available on Amazon as paperbacks and on Kindle as eBooks.

About El Amarna Publishing

El Amarna Publishing is dedicated to producing books, monographs, and e-books for an eclectic but discerning reading audience who enjoy the pursuit of leading edge ideas and philosophies.

We appreciate quality fiction and nonfiction of all genres. For example, we will consider publishing books on history or historical fiction; true detective stories or mysteries; science or science fiction; works on the American West or western novels; true ghost stories or paranormal fiction; women's literature or unique romantic fiction; and any other types of literature as long as the ideas presented are forward thinking and the writing is high quality.

We also plan to publish works of humor; unusual cookbooks; volumes on art, dance, drama, music, and poetry, as well as on the artists who create these things. We will promote well-researched approaches to mythology, symbolism, dreams, esoteric astrology, and divining, as well as metaphysics, mysticism, and magic; and we value the work of creative visionaries in all fields, especially in the categories of comparative religion, interfaith spirituality, personal growth, cultural history, humanistic psychology, and futurism.

Please visit our website, www.ElAmarnaPublishing.com, for submission requirements.

About El Annzar Publishing

www.ingramcontent.com/pod-product-compliance
Lightning Source LLC
Chambersburg PA
CBHW032117280326
41933CB00009B/873